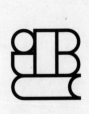

Prisons and AIDS

Prisons and AIDS

A Public Health Challenge

Ronald L. Braithwaite
Theodore M. Hammett
Robert M. Mayberry

Foreword by James W. Curran
Afterword by James S. Jackson

Jossey-Bass Publishers • San Francisco

Substantial discounts on bulk quantities of Jossey-Bass books are available to
corporations, professional associations, and other organizations. For details and
discount information, contact the special sales department at Jossey-Bass Inc.,
Publishers (415) 433–1740; Fax (800) 605–2665.

For sales outside the United States, please contact your local Simon & Schuster
International Office.

 Manufactured in the United States of America on Lyons Falls Pathfinder
Tradebook. This paper is acid-free and 100 percent totally chlorine-free.

Library of Congress Cataloging-in-Publication Data

Braithwaite, Ronald L.
    Prisons and AIDS: a public health challenge/Ronald L. Braithwaite, Theodore M.
    Hammett, Robert M. Mayberry; foreword by James W. Curran; afterword by James
    S. Jackson.
        p. cm.—(The Jossey-Bass health series)
    Includes bibliographical references and index.
    ISBN 0–7879–0308–6 (alk. paper)
    1. AIDS (Disease)—United States. 2. Prisoners—Health and hygiene—United
    States— I. Hammett, Theodore M. II. Mayberry, Robert Morris. III. Title. IV. Series.
    RA644.A25B697 1996
    362.1'969792'008692—dc20   96–22690

FIRST EDITION
HB Printing 10 9 8 7 6 5 4 3 2 1

The Jossey-Bass Health Series

Contents

Contents

List of Tables

Foreword

In the last three centuries, humanity has witnessed spectacular improvements in health and quality of life for vast segments of the world's population. Many improvements in public health have stemmed from scientific advances, pivotal shifts in public health policies and practice, and changes in social policies and practices. Better sanitation methods in communities have been notably effective in dramatically reducing associated infectious diseases. The discovery of antibiotics and vaccines has greatly reduced morbidity and mortality due to bacterial infections, eradicated smallpox, and greatly diminished polio, measles, and rubella in many countries. These scientific achievements have boosted hopes for eradicating deadly and debilitating infectious diseases. The hopes have perhaps been premature; they have also given us false assurance of success.

Shortly after many sounded the death knell for infectious diseases in industrialized countries, in 1981 the first cases of Acquired Immune Deficiency Syndrome (AIDS) were reported in the United States. Over the next decade, the paradigmatic attitude toward AIDS (and other communicable diseases) changed from apathy to panic—the latter due to concerns about the deadly human immunodeficiency virus (HIV) being spread through blood transfusions or casual contact with infected persons. Often public fear led to increased discrimination against persons with HIV—or even those at increased risk of infection.

Many of those at greatest risk in the United States (e.g., gay men, persons with a history of drug use), were no strangers to discrimination. But these attitudes further inhibited the communication and trust needed to establish effective education and prevention efforts. The HIV infection rate among blacks and Hispanics in the United States reinforces the view that HIV/AIDS is a "minority disease" and fosters denial that individual behavior is the major contributor to risk and prevention of HIV infection.

Just as the HIV epidemic has changed our view of infectious disease in society, so also it must transform the paradigm for public health and prevention in prisons and jails. Although, in a very real sense, prisons and jails are seen as a means of social isolation, infections such as HIV and tuberculosis are not so easily isolated. Both infections are potentially fatal, are often acquired before admission, and, if uncontrolled, can spread within the system as well as to others on the outside after the inmate is discharged.

A recent survey indicates that prison inmates are nearly six times more likely than the general population to have AIDS. The CDC reported that 5,279 prisoners had AIDS in 1994. This represents 5.2 cases per 1,000 inmates, while amongst all Americans over age eighteen the rate is 0.9 per 1,000. By the end of 1994, the number of AIDS deaths among inmates (during incarceration) reached 4,558.

Ignoring opportunities for prevention of HIV infection, STDs, and tuberculosis in prisons and jails is a high-risk, short-sighted societal strategy. Everyone knows that unprotected sexual intercourse and injecting drug use occur with some frequency in correctional institutions despite not being condoned. This gap between policy and reality, and the scarcity of resources available for public health interventions in crowded prisons, provides a major challenge.

But perhaps the greatest challenge for public health and correctional health practitioners will involve collaboration on policy formulation and policy implementation responsive to both health promotion and security issues within penal systems. There exists a continuing need for increased research and development in correctional institutions as it relates to effective, culturally sensitive approaches to HIV education and prevention, and to issues regarding transmission while incarcerated.

Prisons and AIDS: A Public Health Challenge represents an important contribution to the field. Its primary goal is to confront the challenges of stimulating a healthier environment through the transfer of education and prevention methods and technologies to prison settings.

July 1996   JAMES W. CURRAN, M.D., M.P.H.
                               Dean
                               Rollins School of Public Health
                               of Emory University

Preface

Prisons and AIDS: A Public Health Challenge evolved from the authors' concern about the many systemic barriers to health promotion and disease prevention programs typical of incarcerated populations. Specifically, access to culturally relevant HIV/AIDS prevention and education programs is more the exception than the rule among correctional institutions. This book is intended to meet the need for a readily accessible resource on selected topics pertinent to engaging social offenders in the design and execution of HIV/AIDS education and prevention programs. The book places emphasis on ethnic minorities, who are disproportionately represented in these institutions and among the general HIV-infected population. While it is not intended to be an exhaustive treatment of all aspects of HIV/AIDS as manifested in prison settings, the book's contents provide information on some of the salient concerns and public health challenges related to sexually transmitted disease and particularly HIV/AIDS.

The book has five purposes:

1. To provide a forum for stimulating discussion on appropriate strategies and models for the prevention of HIV/AIDS within the prison population
2. To document the nature and scope of the HIV/AIDS pandemic among social offenders
3. To offer intervention strategies for addressing this disease from a public health perspective
4. To advance knowledge on policy issues that must be considered by correctional administrators, public policymakers, and academicians training students to assume professional roles in these institutions as health providers and psychosocial support personnel
5. To identify areas for future research and development on HIV/AIDS in correctional settings

The book is intended for persons in several different audiences:

Public health
Health education
Epidemiology
Psychology
Criminology
Sociology
Public administration
Medical sociology
Anthropology
Criminal justice
Correctional rehabilitation
Community health
Nursing
Allied health
Human service
Social policy
Social welfare

Overview of the Contents

Chapter One, "Inmates, HIV, and AIDS: An Overview," sets the stage by providing an overview of the problem confronted by inmates across different types of correctional facilities. This chapter is based on a series of National Institute of Justice (NIJ) and Centers for Disease Control and Prevention (CDC) surveys for the period 1985–1994. The chapter addresses patterns of AIDS cases among adult inmates and confined juveniles, HIV seroprevalence rates, and evidence regarding HIV transmission in adult correctional facilities and juvenile facilities.

Chapter Two, "AIDS and Ethnic Minority Inmates," discusses the well-known problem of ethnic minorities being disproportionately represented in correctional facilities across the United States. Historic discrimination, low socioeconomic status, lack of opportunity, lack of targeted social marketing, and other social forces negatively impact these ethnic groups and are underlying conditions of high-risk behavior. These issues are delineated in this chapter, with emphasis on strategies for developing culturally sensitive HIV/AIDS prevention programs in correctional settings.

Chapter Three, "An Analysis of Current Educational and Prevention Efforts," provides an extensive literature review and meta-analysis of epidemiologic studies of HIV/AIDS in correctional settings, with a specific focus on ethnically diverse populations. The emphasis is on assessment of HIV seroprevalence, knowledge, and risk behavior. A typology for capturing the salient factors across studies is described and analyzed with recommendations and implications for future research on HIV risk reduction.

Chapter Four, "Prevention and Juvenile Offenders," explores policies and programs on HIV and sexually transmitted disease (STD) education/prevention, HIV and STD testing and disclosure, and housing. Issues peculiar to the juvenile setting, such as parental notification, are also addressed.

Chapter Five, "Policy Response to a Public Health Opportunity," explores patterns of policy response in the areas of HIV education/prevention, HIV precautionary and preventive measures, HIV testing and disclosure policies, housing and correctional management of inmates with HIV disease, medical care and psychosocial services, and discharge planning and post-release services within adult correctional facilities.

Chapter Six, "A Report from the Frontline: Four Case Studies," represents a synthesis of interviews and surveys of racial/ethnic social offenders from a medium-security state medical penal institution, an inner-city juvenile detention system, a female adult county jail system, and a rural boot camp facility. Risk behaviors prior to incarceration and current practices are discussed. Issues about sexuality include sexual self-identification, number of encounters, number of sexual partners on first encounter, number of different partners, types of sexual contact (consensual, quasi-consensual, forced), use of condoms by respondents and respondents' partners, and assessment of amount of sexual activity among inmates in the four facilities. Results regarding drug use, needle sharing, and tattooing behaviors are also reported in this chapter.

Chapter Seven, "Prison Personnel: Gatekeepers to Education and Prevention," addresses the myriad challenges faced by correctional administrators and staff related to HIV education and prevention programming and staff perceptions about HIV/AIDS issues.

Chapter Eight, "Legal and Legislative Issues," details case law and legislation regarding mandatory testing, HIV transmission, confidentiality, segregation, access to correctional programs, adequacy of medical care, and indictment and sentencing of persons with HIV/AIDS. The legal ramifications of inmates' biting and spitting on correctional staff are also discussed.

Chapter Nine, "Worldwide Policies and Practices," presents a synopsis of HIV/AIDS programs and practices in foreign correctional institutions. Emphasis is placed on the nature of research activity and educational intervention programs designed to prevent HIV/AIDS during and after incarceration.

Chapter Ten, "The Public Health Challenge," details HIV/AIDS programmatic and policy areas for consideration by both correctional officials and public health officials.

The book closes with "A Guide to Education and Prevention Resources." It details and enumerates existing HIV/AIDS prevention resources available to those serving incarcerated social offenders prior to and upon their release from correctional settings. Resources identified include materials for curriculum development, print and audiovisual products, and lists of advocacy organizations concerned with HIV/AIDS prevention in correctional settings.

Acknowledgments

The book is the result of many dedicated persons' believing in the need to combat the HIV/AIDS pandemic. A debt of gratitude is due our families, who provided encouragement and support during the various stages of this project. We are especially thankful to the many students at the Rollins School of Public Health of Emory University, who provided research assistance during the final stages of this effort. They include Sue Bath, Corliss Heath, Navvab Pike, Michael Daniels, Xianghong Mao, Clark Denny, Tammy Woodring, James Griffin, Torrence Stephens, Elgin Andrews, and Tameika Glover. Our appreciation for professional and technical assistance is extended to the following colleagues: James Griffin, Torrence Stephens, Ken Resnicow, Dazon Dixon, and Stephen Thomas. Special thanks is given to Dr. Sandra E. Taylor for editing final drafts of the chapters. The efforts of the CDC prison research study team were extremely helpful during the data-gathering phase related to Chapters Six and Seven. The team included Benita Harris, Goodman Obot, Juarlyn Gaiter, Melanie Duckworth, Dennis Jarvis, Jo Valentine, Henry Murdaugh, William Blackman, Dannielle Lentine, Robert Morris, Charles Baker, Susan Huscroft, Algea Harrison, Jo Anne Holbert, Scott Cozza, Regene Polk, Wayne Johnson, and Jill Lester. A special thanks goes to Dorothy Triplett for her support; she was especially instrumental in facilitating the sustained funding for this initiative. We thank Cheri Crawford and Virginia Baldau at the National Institute of Justice, Sandy Kerr and Steve Jones at the Centers for Disease Control and Prevention, and literally hundreds of correctional administrators, health services staff, and others who completed the questionnaires and participated in site visits for assistance with and support of surveys on which Chapters One, Four, Five, and Eight are largely based.

The following Abt Associates staff also contributed writing, research, information, and assistance in the course of the series of national studies of HIV/AIDS in correctional facilities that was sponsored by NIJ and CDC. Rebecca Widom contributed substantially to Chapter Four; Joel Epstein contributed substantially to Chapter Eight; Lynne Harrold directed the survey data collection for a number of years. Others at Abt Associates deserving acknowledgment include Santiago Sifre, Tammy Enos, David Deal, Mary-Ellen Perry, Wendy Sanderson, Karen Minich, and Winn Sinclair.

We are also grateful to Simone Ladson and Alice Henderson, who prepared this manuscript for the publisher. Lastly, we express sincere appreciation to Rebecca McGovern at Jossey-Bass. Without her untiring efforts, this book would not exist.

July 1996   RONALD L. BRAITHWAITE
                                       Atlanta, Georgia
                                       THEODORE M. HAMMETT
                                       Cambridge, Massachusetts
                                       ROBERT M. MAYBERRY
                                       Atlanta, Georgia

To HIV/AIDS educators throughout the world

The Authors

Ronald L. Braithwaite, Ph.D., is an associate professor at the Rollins School of Public Health of Emory University and adjunct associate professor in the department of community health and preventive medicine at Morehouse School of Medicine, where he formerly directed a health promotion resource center. He received his B.A. and M.S. from Southern Illinois University in sociology and rehabilitation, respectively. He received the Ph.D. degree from Michigan State University in educational psychology in 1974. He has done postdoctoral studies at Howard University, Yale University, and the University of Michigan (School of Public Health and Institute for Social Research). He has conducted program evaluation of educational, health, and human service programs using several contemporary models for program evaluation.

Braithwaite has taught research design, statistics, program evaluation, test and measurement, community organization, and minority health at the graduate level to nursing, medical, and public health students. He is widely published in education and health journals; he recently co-edited *Health Issues in the Black Community* (1992, Jossey-Bass). His work in community organization and development has gained national attention. He has also served as principal investigator evaluating HIV/AIDS education and prevention programs in correctional settings for a grant funded by the Centers for Disease Control and Prevention and the Association of Schools of Public Health.

Currently he serves as principal investigator and co-principal investigator for two high-risk youth demonstration grants from the Center for Substance Abuse Prevention. Additionally he is the principal investigator for a community-based public health practice partnership funded by the Health Resources and Services Administration. He has served as a consultant to numerous federal, state, and private organizations.

Theodore M. Hammett, Ph.D., is a vice president at Abt Associates, Inc., a leading policy research firm with headquarters in Cambridge, Massachusetts. In his seventeen years with Abt Associates, Hammett has focused on work in public health, corrections, and criminal justice. Since 1985, he has directed a series of eight national studies of HIV/AIDS in correctional facilities under the joint sponsorship of the National Institute of Justice, U.S. Department of Justice, and the Centers for Disease Control and Prevention. He has also published numerous reports and articles on HIV/AIDS, tuberculosis, and STDs as they affect criminal justice agencies and offender populations.

Hammett also directed a multisite demonstration and evaluation of an HIV prevention program for female commercial sex workers and sexual partners of injection drug users, funded by the National Institute on Drug Abuse. He has spoken before numerous national and international conferences, testified before the National Commission on AIDS, and participated in an invited consultation on HIV/AIDS in prisons at the World Health Organization in Geneva.

Robert M. Mayberry, M.P.H., Ph.D., currently serves as the director of the Morehouse Medical Treatment Effectiveness Center (MMEDTEC) and an associate clinical professor in the department of community health and preventive medicine at the Morehouse School of Medicine. He is responsible for research development in medical-effective (patient outcomes) research targeting African American populations. He earned a B.A. and an M.S. in biology from Berea College and Alabama A & M University, respectively. He received his M.P.H. and Ph.D. in epidemiology from the University of California at Berkeley. A former visiting professor at the Rollins School of Public Health of Emory University, Mayberry has held positions as senior epidemiologist in the director's office, associate director for minority health at the Centers for Disease Control and Prevention; assistant dean at the Graduate School of the University of South Carolina; and assistant professor in the department of epidemiology and biostatistics in the School of Public Health at the University of South Carolina.

Mayberry's areas of specialization are cancer epidemiology (etiologic investigations of racial/ethnic variations in cancer incidence and survival), treatment effectiveness (patient outcome) research with a focus on African American populations (prenatal care content, low birth weight, and infant mortality; variations in health care services and health outcomes by race/ethnicity), and epidemiologic principles and methods in program planning and evaluation. Having served and chaired many local and state commissions and task forces, he is active in local, state, and national health organizations, with membership in the American Public Health Association, the Society for Epidemiologic Research, the American Statistical Association, and the Association of Health Services Research. He was the founder and first president of the South Carolina Coalition for Public Health.

Chapter One

Inmates, HIV, and AIDS
An Overview

In addition to the already daunting problems posed by severe crowding and fiscal stringency, today's correctional administrators and health care professionals working in prisons and jails must deal with an increasingly ill, troubled, and "graying" inmate population. HIV/AIDS is but one facet of a complex of health and psychosocial problems that are becoming increasingly common among inmates, including tuberculosis, sexually transmitted diseases, substance abuse, and mental illness.

These problems—which are significantly associated with high-risk sexual activity, poverty, homelessness, and poor access to preventive and primary health care—pose difficult programmatic and fiscal challenges for administrators and staff of prison and jail systems. Ironically, these problems also offer opportunities for public health agencies, community-based organizations, and correctional systems to address and help improve the health of a particularly underserved and vulnerable segment of the population. Administrators, health, and mental health workers in prisons and jails have a unique opportunity to assist inmates—who are literally a "captive audience" and thus at least logistically easier to reach than similar at-risk populations in the community—with health care, prevention, education, and substance abuse treatment (Glaser & Greifinger, 1993). Better HIV/AIDS, TB, and STDs (sexually transmitted diseases) prevention programs and medical care in prisons and jails will also benefit the larger society, since the vast majority of inmates return to the community.

To date, providers of correctional health care and prevention services have not fully taken advantage of the public health opportunity available to them. Nor have corrections, public health, and community-based organizations yet forged the partnerships needed to exploit this opportunity with effectiveness and efficiency. However, it remains a significant opportunity that can be addressed by carefully designed programs and dedicated staff (Polonsky et al., 1994; Glaser & Greifinger, 1993; Snider, Thorburn, Warren, & Dowdle, 1993).

In the words of the medical director of the Federal Bureau of Prisons, the correctional response to these challenges and opportunities requires a "balancing of the dual missions of custody and care" (Moritsugu, 1993). Because of the often differing perspectives and priorities between correctional officials and health care workers, such a balance is, in itself, a challenge to achieve (Anno, 1991).

This chapter presents the most up-to-date statistics available on HIV/AIDS in adult prisons and jails and juvenile facilities. These data are drawn from the eighth in a series of national surveys, jointly sponsored by the Centers for Disease Control and Prevention and the National Institute of Justice (U.S. Department of Justice) and conducted between May and December 1994 (Hammett et al., 1995; Widom & Hammett, 1996). As in previous years of the survey, responses were received from all fifty state correctional systems and the Federal Bureau of Prisons. Twenty-nine large city and county jail systems also responded to the 1994 NIJ/CDC survey. In an effort to assess the extent to which individual facilities comply with or depart from policies established by systems' central offices, the 1994 survey for the first time included a validation study in which an abbreviated version of the instrument (covering only key policy areas) was sent to a sample of fifty facilities in fourteen state systems and the Federal Bureau of Prisons. Forty-one state juvenile systems responded to the survey, as did thirty-two large city/county juvenile detention centers.

AIDS Cases Among Adult Inmates

A cumulative total of 11,565 AIDS cases had been reported among inmates in U.S. federal, state, and larger city/county correctional systems as of November 1992, when the seventh NIJ/CDC survey was completed (Hammett, Harrold, Gross, & Epstein, 1994). (As discussed below, it was not possible to calculate cumulative totals based on the eighth survey, conducted in 1994.) This figure represents cumulative totals since the beginning of the epidemic. Of these cases, 8,525 occurred among inmates of forty-eight state prison systems (two state systems reported no cases) and the Federal Bureau of Prisons. Three thousand forty (3,040) cases were reported by thirty-one city/county jail systems.

The cumulative figures require some qualification. The NIJ/CDC survey is not exhaustive of city/county jail systems, and the participating jail systems have varied slightly from year to year. Some components of the data necessary to calculate cumulative totals (current cases, cases among released individuals, and deaths while in custody) were not available from every jurisdiction for every year of the survey. Therefore, some components of the totals have been estimated based on prior years' reports. However, these estimates have always been made conservatively. Collectively, the conservative estimation of components, the inexhaustive scope of the survey, and the undercounting in some correctional systems that has come to light over time suggest that the cumulative total figures be considered minimum estimates of the cumulative incidence of AIDS among U.S. inmates through 1993. Based on this minimum estimate, at least 4.6 percent of the U.S. cases of AIDS through 1993 occurred among inmates.

Table 1.1 shows that the rate of increase in cumulative total correctional cases over the two years since the previous survey is 66 percent. Assuming the growth was spread evenly over the two years, the annual rate of increase was about 33 percent for each of the last three years. The rate of increase in correctional cases between 1990 and 1992 (66 percent) was slightly above that in the total U.S. population (64 percent) for the same period.

Beginning with the 1994 NIJ/CDC survey, the cumulative total figure could no longer be calculated because of increasing levels of missing data and consequent increasing uncertainty. In the 1994 survey, over half of the correctional systems were unable to provide figures for inmates released with HIV/AIDS, always the most problematic component to obtain. This seemed an unacceptably high level of missing data. By contrast, almost all systems were able to

Table 1.1. Cumulative Total AIDS Cases Among Correctional Inmates and the Population at Large, United States, 1985–1992.

	Correctional Cases[a]		Cases in Total U.S. Population[b]	
	n	% Increase from Preceding Year[c]	n	% Increase from Preceding Year[d]
November 1985	766	n/a	14,519	n/a
October 1986	1,232	61 %	26,002	79 %
October 1987	1,964	59	41,770	61
October 1988[e]	3,136	60	73,621	76
October 1989[f]	5,411	72	110,333	50
October 1990[g]	6,985	29	152,231	38
November 1992 –March 1993[h]	11,565	66	249,199	64

[a] The figures in this and other tables represent inmate AIDS cases in the federal prison system, all fifty state prison systems, and a sample of from twenty-eight to thirty-seven city and county jail systems (depending on the year of the NIJ survey).

[b] Adult/adolescent cases only. Pediatric cases excluded.

[c] In most cases, the column presents the difference between the number of cases in the given year and the number in the prior year. The exception is November 1992 through March 1993.

[d] As with the correctional cases, the percent increase reflects the change from the preceding survey. In most cases, this is a one-year interval. However, the percent increase for November 1992 through March 1993 reflects a two-year interval.

[e] Figures for 1988 include twenty-eight city/county jail systems.

[f] Figures for 1989 include thirty-two city/county jail systems.

[g] Figures for 1990 include twenty-seven city/county jail systems.

[h] Figures for 1992 include thirty-one city/county jail systems.

n/a = not available.

Sources: CDC, *AIDS Weekly Surveillance Reports* (United States, Nov. 4, 1985, Oct. 5, 1986, Oct. 5, 1987, Oct. 3, 1988); CDC, *HIV/AIDS Surveillance Report,* Nov. 1990, Feb. 1993 (cases reported through 1992); NIJ/CDC questionnaire responses.

provide figures for current cases and deaths. It was therefore decided to discontinue the cumulative total calculation and present only current cases and deaths.

AIDS Deaths Among Adult Inmates

While it is unfortunate to break the time series based on cumulative total AIDS cases, a time series on inmate deaths can be substituted. This time series for inmates can be compared to the equivalent time series in the total U.S. population, as was previously done with the cumulative case totals. This comparison is presented in Table 1.2. In 1992, 1993, and 1994, cumulative inmate AIDS deaths increased 32 percent, while cumulative AIDS deaths in the total population increased 42 percent. Since 1985, inmate AIDS deaths have increased by 1,311 percent, while AIDS deaths in the U.S. population increased by 2,904 percent, more than twice as large an increase.

Table 1.2 shows that 4,588 inmates in the reporting correctional systems had died of HIV/AIDS as of December 1994, when the survey was completed. This should not be considered an absolutely accurate count, since the survey was not exhaustive of all correctional systems and underreporting may have occurred in participating systems. However, the figure represents 2 percent of the cumulative total HIV/AIDS deaths reported in the United States through June 1994 (240,323). Twenty-one percent of reported inmate HIV/AIDS deaths occurred since the 1992 NIJ/CDC survey.

The distribution of cumulative total HIV/AIDS deaths across correctional systems is quite uneven. Forty-three state/federal systems reported 3,870 total deaths. Six state/federal systems reported more than 100 inmate HIV/AIDS deaths, and seven systems reported more than 50 deaths. The NIJ/CDC survey captures data from all state correctional systems and the Federal Bureau of Prisons, but it includes only a relatively small number of city/county jail systems. In 1994, twenty-nine jail systems submitted responses. The sample includes the largest U.S. jail systems but omits many others of substantial size. In 1994, seventeen city/county jail systems in the NIJ/CDC survey reported a total of 718 inmate HIV/AIDS deaths. Only one of the jail systems reported more than

Table 1.2. Cumulative Total AIDS Cases Among Correctional Inmates and the Population at Large, U.S., 1985–1994.

	Cumulative Correctional Cases[a]		Cumulative Deaths in Total U.S. Population[b]	
	n	% Increase from Preceding Year	n	% Increase from Preceding Year
November 1985	325	n/a	8,000	n/a
October 1986	533	64 %	16,500	106 %
October 1987	865	62	24,412	48
October 1988	1,306	51	42,142	73
October 1989	1,423	9	65,467	55
October 1990	2,504	76	94,375	44
November 1992	3,474	39	169,623	80
December 1994	4,588	32	240,323	42

[a] The figures in this table represent inmate AIDS deaths in the federal prison system, all fifty state prison systems, and a sample of twenty-eight to thirty-seven large city and county jail systems (depending on the year of the survey).

[b] Adult/adolescent cases only. Pediatric cases excluded.

n/a = not available.

Sources: CDC, *AIDS Weekly Surveillance Reports* (United States, Nov. 4, 1985, Oct. 5, 1986, Oct. 5, 1987, Oct. 3, 1988); CDC, *HIV/AIDS Surveillance Report,* Nov. 1989, Nov. 1990, Feb. 1993 (cases reported through 1992), 1994 midyear edition (cases reported through June 1994); NIJ/CDC questionnaire responses.

100 inmate deaths from HIV/AIDS, one reported 2,650 deaths, and five reported 1,125 deaths.

Additional data on HIV/AIDS deaths in jails come from the annual survey of jails conducted by the Bureau of Justice Statistics (BJS), U.S. Department of Justice. The most recently available statistics, for 1992, cover 503 jurisdictions with inmate populations in excess of 100. Thirty-seven of these jurisdictions with "large jail populations" reported 107 inmate AIDS deaths during 1992. This represents 24 percent of the 445 total inmate deaths reported to the BJS jail survey by these jurisdictions in 1992 (Bureau of Justice Statistics, 1993). The regional distribution of total inmate

HIV/AIDS deaths is also uneven, with the most deaths in the Middle Atlantic region (principally New York and New Jersey).

Current AIDS Cases Among Adult Inmates

In 1994, forty-seven state and federal prison systems reported 4,827 current cases, an increase of 59 percent over the 1992–1993 survey. This increase is less steep than might be expected, given the change in the AIDS case definition that went into effect at the start of 1993. This may result from less aggressive testing and diagnostic services and less complete reporting of cases in correctional facilities than in the outside community. State and federal prison systems reported a range of zero percent to 2.4 percent of inmates having AIDS diagnoses. Jail systems reported 0–1.4 percent of inmates having AIDS diagnoses.

Twenty-three city/county jail systems reported 452 current AIDS cases in 1994, an increase of 14 percent from 1992–1993. The distribution is quite uneven among state/federal systems, with 22 percent of the systems reporting 83 percent of current cases. Fourteen percent of city/county systems reported 44 percent of current cases, a somewhat more even distribution.

AIDS Incidence Rates Among Adult Inmates

The annual AIDS incidence rate in the total U.S. population in 1994 was 31 cases per 100,000 population. This was up sharply from 18 in 1992 due to the revised AIDS case definition. State incidence rates ranged from three cases per 100,000 in North Dakota to 82 cases per 100,000 in New York. Rates in metropolitan areas with populations in excess of 500,000 ranged from five in Ann Arbor, Michigan, to 254 in Washington, D.C. (Centers for Disease Control and Prevention, 1994b).

AIDS incidence rates are significantly higher among correctional inmates than in the total population. This is because of the high concentrations in correctional populations of persons with risk factors for HIV infection. Incidence rates in correctional systems vary widely, reflecting the uneven distribution of actual cases, as well as divergent diagnostic and reporting practices across systems. In state/federal systems in 1994, the aggregate AIDS incidence rate (based on the total cases and the total inmate populations across all systems) was 518 cases per 100,000, up from 362 cases in 1992.[1] The median incidence rate for state/federal prison systems was 186 AIDS cases per 100,000 inmates in 1994, with a range of zero to 2,375 cases.

The aggregate incidence rate for reporting city/county jail systems was 706 cases per 100,000 inmates in 1994. The median incidence rate was 289 cases, with a range of zero to 1,416 cases. However, the high turnover rates of jail inmates make these incidence rates difficult to interpret.

HIV Seroprevalence Among Adult Inmates

Mandatory screening (mandatory, identity-linked testing of all incoming, current, or about-to-be-released inmates) and blinded epidemiologic studies both capture populations uninfluenced by selection biases. Therefore, HIV seropositivity rates based on these two methods are probably the most reliable estimates of HIV seroprevalence among correctional inmates. Statistics submitted by respondents to the NIJ/CDC surveys based on mandatory screening and blinded studies show that HIV seroprevalence rates vary widely from system to system. Most systems continue to have rates of 1 percent or below, while a few systems have rates as high as 20–26 percent (females in New York State and New York City). Jurisdictions with rates of inmate HIV seropositivity of over 5 percent based on mandatory screening or blinded studies include New Jersey, Massachusetts, Florida, Cook County (Chicago), and Illinois (females only). Systems with rates of 2–5 percent include California, Texas, Georgia, North Carolina, and King County (Seattle).

In most systems with data available for more than one period, HIV seroprevalence rates are most often stable or, in a few cases, declining. Reductions in HIV seroprevalence based on blinded studies occurred in New York State (among males, from 17 percent in 1987–1988 to 15 percent in 1990 [$p = .01$] and 11.5 percent in 1992 [$p = .01$]) and Florida (among females, from 24 percent in 1992 to 11 percent in 1993). Based on mandatory testing programs, HIV seroprevalence dropped from 2.4 percent to 1.4 percent from 1990–1992 to 1994 in Nevada, and among females in New Hampshire from 7 percent in 1989–1990 to 3 percent in 1992 and 2 percent in 1993. There were a few increases in HIV seroprevalence. Rates among incoming male inmates in New Hampshire increased from 0.5 percent in 1989–1990 to 1.3 percent in 1992 and 2.2 percent in 1993. In Louisiana, based on blinded studies, HIV seroprevalence among males rose from 0.3 percent in 1990–1991 to 1.9 percent in 1992–1994.

Comparisons of HIV seropositivity rates from mandatory screening or blinded studies on the one hand and voluntary testing on the other are mixed. In New York State, blinded studies of incoming male and female inmates found higher rates of HIV seropositivity than did on-request testing (15 percent versus 7.5 percent for males, 20 percent versus 13.4 percent for females) (LaChance-McCullough, Tesoriero, Sorin, & Lee, 1993; LaChance-McCullough, Tesoriero, Sorin, & Stern, 1994). Similarly, in Massachusetts, HIV seroprevalence rates from a blinded study (7 percent for males and 13 percent for females) were higher than seropositivity rates from voluntary testing (2 percent for males and 5 percent for females). These discrepancies may reflect reluctance on the part of persons who know they are at risk to "get the bad news" and/or fear that their HIV status will be disclosed and lead to discrimination or mistreatment. HIV seropositivity rates were higher based on voluntary testing than on blinded studies in Rhode Island (both males and females), Florida (females only; male rates were similar), Rhode Island, and Washington (males only; female rates were similar). In these jurisdictions, inmates who believed they were at elevated risk were, for whatever reason, more willing to come forward for testing.

HIV seroprevalence is often higher among female inmates than among male inmates. This pattern seems most common in the Northeast, where New York City, New York State, New Jersey, Massachusetts, Connecticut, and Rhode Island all report higher rates for females than males. This may be due to the high prevalence of injection drug use and crack use among female inmates in these states. Elsewhere, HIV seroprevalence is higher among females than among males in Florida, Illinois, Cook County (Chicago), Nevada, California, and Washington State.

Characteristics of Adult Inmates with HIV/AIDS

The vast majority of inmate AIDS deaths and current AIDS cases continue to occur among men. Ninety-six percent of cumulative AIDS deaths and 91 percent of current inmate AIDS cases in 1994 were among males. Aggregate AIDS incidence rates in state/federal systems were 464 cases per 100,000 among men and 705 cases among women. In responding city/county jail systems, the rates were 342 cases per 100,000 among men and 201 cases among women. As discussed above, HIV seroprevalence is very often higher among female than male inmates.

Moreover, incarceration rates are rising faster among women than men, and women in prisons and jails are more likely to be drug users than are male inmates. Economic dependency, injection drug use, crack use, and associated increases in unsafe sexual practices (for example, exchanging sex for drugs and/or money) have placed many women at elevated risk for HIV/AIDS. Recent studies of incarcerated women in New York and Massachusetts confirm the correlates of high rates of HIV infection. In a New York study of 216 women who agreed to voluntary testing (29, or 13 percent, of whom were HIV seropositive), injection drug use was the most significant predictor of HIV seropositivity, with drug injection in a shooting gallery further increasing the likelihood of being HIV seropositive (LaChance-McCullough et al., 1993; LaChance-McCullough et al., 1994).

A study of eighty-seven women recruited through the infectious disease clinic at Massachusetts Correctional Institution, Framingham (70 percent of whom were HIV seropositive), explored a broader range of potential correlates than did the New York study. The Massachusetts study found that injection drug use, commercial sex work, a history of childhood sexual abuse, and a history of genital or anal warts were all predictive of HIV seropositivity. Perhaps the most important finding of this study is the strong association between sexual abuse and risk-taking behaviors related to HIV (Stevens et al., 1995). These findings indicate the importance of incorporating counseling for survivors of sexual abuse in HIV prevention programs for women.

Different correctional systems supplied various combinations of statistics regarding race and ethnicity of inmates with AIDS to the 1994 NIJ/CDC survey. Combining these statistics reveals the median racial/ethnic breakdowns of AIDS cases in responding state/federal systems as 43 percent black, 38 percent white, and 13 percent Hispanic. This compares with the distribution among total cumulative AIDS cases in the U.S. population of 50 percent white,

32 percent black, and 17 percent Hispanic. The disproportion in the total U.S. population is thus primarily between whites and blacks. The difference is even more striking in city/county systems, where the median distributions are 58 percent black, 15 percent white, and 14 percent Hispanic. Other data also reveal disproportional distributions of cases by racial and ethnic groups, but with some differences. Of cases reported in the total New York State population through September 1995, 31 percent were among whites, 40 percent among blacks, and 29 percent among Hispanics. Among New York State inmate cases, 12 percent were among whites, 41 percent among blacks, and 47 percent among Hispanics. The most striking difference in these New York State figures is the overrepresentation of Hispanics among inmates with AIDS. This may reflect the large Puerto Rican component of the Hispanic inmate population; this population has particularly high rates of HIV infection due to the movement of injection drug users back and forth between Puerto Rico and New York City communities, reinforcing the already high levels of HIV infection in these communities.

Although the NIJ/CDC survey does not seek breakdowns of AIDS cases by exposure categories because previous efforts to obtain this information were largely unsuccessful, data from other sources indicate that injection drug use is probably the most common exposure category in inmate AIDS cases. Among New York State inmate cases reported through March 1994, 93 percent were attributed to injection drug use. Studies in New York City and Maryland have also shown injection drug use to be the primary inmate exposure category (Vlahov et al., 1989; Weisfuse et al., 1991). Nationwide HIV testing data suggest increasing rates of infections due to heterosexual contact and other unprotected sex, especially among women. These patterns may begin to be reflected in correctional populations.

HIV Transmission Among Adult Correctional Inmates

HIV transmission among correctional inmates remains a matter of serious concern. Indisputably, sex, injection drug use, and tattooing are occurring in prisons and jails regardless of prohibitions against all of these activities. Condoms are not officially available to inmates in most correctional systems. In the absence of condoms, inmates may use and reuse such expedients as fingers cut from latex surgical gloves (Mahon, 1994a).

Rape and other forms of nonconsensual sex are particularly serious issues demanding serious responses from correctional systems, independently of the issue of HIV transmission. While there is little systematic data on the incidence of rape behind bars, one advocate has asserted that 131,000 adult males are sexually victimized in correctional facilities each year (Donaldson, 1994; Dumond, 1992). In the spring of 1994, a series of investigative articles on rape in Massachusetts prisons prompted the state's Department of Correction to institute new procedures for identifying and investigating alleged rapes. This included training for all correctional officers, counselors, and medical staff (Sennott, 1994a, 1994b). Some members of the Massachusetts legislature and others have called for mandatory HIV testing as a response to the revelations regarding prison rape. In reality, however, rape and HIV are separate issues requiring independent responses (Hammett, 1994).

Research from Britain suggests that injection drug use is less common in prisons than on the outside but considerably more risky, because the very shortage of needles that reduces prevalence of use also increases sharing. Moreover, risk is exacerbated by inmates' often limited understanding of "sharing." In reality, sharing includes not only passing needles among people, but also using needles and syringes that have been used by persons not present, and perhaps not properly cleaned; sharing injection solutions (as in "backloading" and "frontloading"); and sharing containers, cotton, and other paraphernalia (Turnbull, Stimson, & Stilwell, 1994). When needles are not available, pieces of pens and light bulbs are sometimes used by inmates to inject drugs (Mahon, 1994a).

Tattooing is a common practice in prisons and jails. Given the shortage of sterile needles, it is often done with guitar strings and other expedient materials. In tattooing, sharing of the needle (or needle substitute), ink, and string used to transmit the ink may pose risks for HIV transmission (staff at Federal Bureau of Prisons, Metropolitan Correctional Center, Miami, personal communications, Nov. 12, 1994; staff at Northwest State Correctional Center, Swanton, Vermont, Nov. 8, 1994). The only controlled study to date of HIV transmission in correctional facilities was carried out among male inmates in the Illinois Department of Corrections between 1988 and 1990. Of almost 2,400 inmates HIV seronegative on entry to the system (in an attempt to exclude "window period" infections, only inmates who had spent at least three months in a county jail prior to entering the state system were eligible for the study), seven had documented HIV seroconversions after one year of incarceration. This represents an annual incidence rate of 0.3 percent (Castro et al., 1994). Several other U.S. studies with varying methodologies involving baseline and follow-up testing have found annual seroconversion rates of less than 1 percent (Horsburgh, Jarvis, McArther, Ignacio, & Stock, 1990). While these are low rates, they nevertheless demonstrate that transmission has occurred and, when applied to total inmate populations, results in nontrivial numbers of in-prison HIV infections. Based on a model developed by researchers in Australia, annual HIV seroconversion rates among injection drug users in prison may range from 1.7 percent to 3.3 percent, depending on the assumed frequency of shared injections (Dolan, Kaplan, Wodak, Hall, & Gaughwin, 1994).

Several other studies in the United States and Australia have identified cases of HIV infection by testing inmates continuously incarcerated since before the supposed appearance of HIV in the population (Dolan, Hall, Wodak, & Gaughwin, 1994). The American study comes from the Florida State correctional system, where 87 of 556 inmates continuously incarcerated since 1977 had been voluntarily tested for HIV antibody and 18 were positive. This represents a seropositivity rate of 21 percent on the basis of the number tested (Mutter, Grimes, & Labarthe, 1994). This is quite a high rate. However, it is important to note that it may represent a self-selected sample of those who sought testing because they felt at risk for HIV infection due to their behaviors in prison. In any case, only 16 percent of those continuously incarcerated since 1977 were tested. Annual HIV seroconversion rates based on total numbers of inmates susceptible (that is, entering seronegative) and years of potential exposure would no doubt be much lower. The article does not present the data necessary to calculate annual seroconversion rates for the entire Florida inmate population. In general, it is equally important to avoid understating and, as the Florida article seems to do, overstating the problem of HIV transmission in correctional facilities. Finally, a Scottish study found evidence of HIV acquisition among prisoners who admitted to injecting drugs while in prison (Taylor et al., 1995).

AIDS Cases Among Confined Juveniles

For the first time in 1994, the NIJ/CDC survey covered juvenile systems. A cumulative total of sixty juveniles with AIDS was reported (fifty boys and ten girls, fifty-four in state and six in city/county systems). Cumulative totals include cases among juveniles currently confined, those who have been released, and those who have died while confined. In the seventy-three juvenile systems responding to the NIJ/CDC survey, there were only four currently confined juveniles with AIDS: three state systems and one city/county detention center each reported having one confined boy with AIDS. No responding systems reported any currently confined girls with AIDS. Respondents reported that a total of four juveniles (two in state systems and two in city/county systems, three boys and one girl) had died from AIDS while confined.

Although rates of HIV disease are not currently very high among adolescents, other sexually transmitted diseases are more prevalent, which indicates that adolescents are at risk for HIV infection, and that more HIV among adolescents in the future is likely. According to recent research, some of the highest rates of gonorrhea during the 1980s were among adolescents 15–19 years old, and rates increased or remained the same among adolescents throughout the 1980s, while rates decreased for other groups. Further, as demonstrated by data from the 1994 NIJ/CDC survey and other sources, confined youth have higher rates of STDs than adolescents in the community, indicating significant risk for HIV among confined youth (Morris, Baker, & Huscroft, 1992; Hammett & Widom, 1996).

HIV Seroprevalence Among Confined Juveniles

Currently, HIV seroprevalence among confined juveniles appears to be low. Blinded epidemiological studies and mass screening both avoid selection bias, thus providing the best estimates of seroprevalence. Blind studies of confined juveniles in Colorado, Texas, and San Bernardino County, California, found no HIV seropositive juveniles in their samples. Studies in Alabama and Illinois found rates of HIV seropositivity of 0.7 percent and 0.1 percent respectively. Screening of all incoming juveniles in New Mexico found no HIV seropositive adolescents among 1,053 boys and 260 girls tested. Similarly, screening in Mississippi found, after testing all incoming juveniles from September 1992 through October 1994, that only one girl was HIV seropositive. All responses from other jurisdictions indicated that HIV testing for other reasons, including testing juveniles upon request and testing pregnant girls, resulted in less than 1 percent seropositivity among confined juveniles.

Although relatively few adolescents with HIV disease have been identified, it is clear that many adolescents engage in HIV-risk activities (including unprotected sexual intercourse and injection drug use). Most research on risk behaviors among adolescents focuses on those in school, and somewhat less on adolescents out of school; very little research has considered confined adolescents. One study found relatively stable levels of sexual activity and drug use among adolescents between 1990 and 1993. However, the same study reported a significant increase in condom use among female and African American adolescents who engage in sexual intercourse, and a decrease in gonorrhea and live births among teenagers 15–19 years old in forty states (Centers for Disease Control and Prevention, 1995). Other research has documented increases in sexual activity, rates of STDs, and unintended pregnancy among high school students since the 1970s, and an increase in HIV infection among high school students since the 1980s (Centers for Disease Control, 1992b). While HIV and STDs are likely to be spreading among adolescents in school, adolescents not in school (including confined juveniles) appear to be at even more serious risk. According to the CDC, out-of-school adolescents aged 14–19 years were significantly more likely than in-school adolescents to report ever having had sexual intercourse (70.1 percent versus 45.4 percent) and to have had four or more sexual partners (36.4 percent versus 14.0 percent) (Centers for Disease Control and Prevention, 1994a). Confined juveniles represent what may be a particularly at-risk subpopulation of adolescents not in school, because of the overrepresentation among them of youths with histories of high-risk behavior and poor access to health care and prevention services.

Conclusion

It is clear that HIV/AIDS is a serious problem among adult correctional inmates and an incipient problem among confined juveniles. Adult prisons and jails and juvenile facilities contain probably the highest concentrations of persons already infected with HIV and individuals with sexual and drug-use related risk factors for HIV to be found anywhere in American society. The vast majority of adult inmates and confined juveniles return to the community, where they may become infected or infect others if they continue or resume their high-risk activities. Finally, high recidivism rates suggest that a substantial population of individuals with HIV infection or risk factors may be cycling in and out of prisons, jails, and juvenile facilities. These facts make it imperative that comprehensive HIV education and prevention programs be implemented and sustained in these facilities.

Note

1. Incidence rates for correctional populations were calculated as follows: current AIDS cases × 100,000/current inmate population. Current cases may be less than the total number of cases reported during the year, thus producing slightly understated incidence rates. However, most correctional systems do not maintain data on AIDS cases by year reported.

Chapter Two

AIDS and
Ethnic Minority Inmates

The health of the United States inmate population should be the concern not only of the correctional institutions that hold them, but also of society as a whole. Currently, AIDS is the leading cause of death among inmates in many correctional facilities across the United States (Pagliaro & Pagliaro, 1992). This statistic is frightening, because at the end of 1994 five million people in the United States were under the control of the criminal justice system, including 1.5 million inmates imprisoned at the federal, state, or local level and 3.5 million on probation or parole (Brien & Harlow, 1995). In fact, the number of people under the control of the criminal justice system continues to rise and will soon surpass the number of students enrolled full-time in four-year colleges or universities, which stands at six million (Brien & Harlow, 1995).

Chapter One documents the serious and growing problem of HIV/AIDS in inmate populations. The AIDS-related health issues of the inmates must concern correctional facilities and noninstitutionalized society, because prisons typically have high turnover rates. Even more importantly, the underlying conditions influencing inmates' high-risk behaviors need to be dealt with by all of society.

This chapter examines ethnic minorities in correctional facilities in light of their disproportionate representation. Additionally, consideration is given to the underlying conditions of high-risk behavior, including historical discrimination, low socioeconomic status, lack of opportunity, lack of targeted social marketing, and other social forces (such as drug addiction). These issues are discussed in this chapter with emphasis on strategies for developing culturally sensitive HIV/AIDS prevention programs in correctional settings.

Representation of Ethnic Minorities in Correctional Facilities

The picture of AIDS in correctional facilities is even grimmer for ethnic minorities. Across the United States, ethnic minorities are disproportionately represented in correctional facilities. In the 1980s, African Americans represented approximately 12 percent of the total population of the United States but accounted for 48 percent of all the inmates in state correctional facilities (Olivero, 1990). From 1990 to 1993, the percentage of black inmates in federal and state prisons rose from 46.5 percent to 50.8 percent, and the percentage of Hispanic inmates nearly doubled from 7.7 percent to 14.3 percent (Brien & Harlow, 1995). For example, in 1991, the Adult Correctional Institute in Rhode Island had a total inmate population of 2,500. There was a disproportionately greater representation of African Americans (greater than fivefold) and Latinos (approximately twofold) compared with the general population in Rhode Island (Dixon et al., 1993). Ethnic minorities are disproportionately represented not only in correctional facilities but also among the AIDS cases in those facilities. For example, in New York State, Hispanics comprise 30 percent of the inmate population but contribute 47 percent of the AIDS cases among inmates (Morse et al., 1990).

Historical Discrimination

Institutionalized Racism

Institutionalized racism in the United States partially explains the overrepresentation of ethnic minorities in various disease categories nationwide (Hutchinson, 1992). Infant deaths, neonatal deaths, and postnatal deaths are twice as high among African Americans compared to whites (Hutchinson, 1992). According to

Konner (1993), an article published in the *New England Journal of Medicine* reports that if the infant mortality rate is removed and life expectancy of a preschool-age child is examined, life expectancies for both boys and girls are worse in Harlem than in Bangladesh. World Bank statistics report that the probability of death between ages fifteen and forty-five for African American males nationally—slightly over 30 percent—is higher than the same statistic for underdeveloped nations such as The Gambia, India, and El Salvador (Konner, 1993). Research suggests that African Americans generally have less access to health care regardless of economic circumstances (Sullivan, 1989). In the United States, there are 35 million uninsured people; African Americans are disproportionately represented within this population (Konner, 1993). In fact, almost one-third of African Americans lack private health insurance, and nearly as many live in states that provide minimal support for Medicaid (Konner, 1993).

Among low-income ethnic minorities, long-term health care is just as unlikely. Health care for poor ethnic minorities is usually done in emergency rooms, where the treatment tends to be expensive and involves long waiting periods, impersonal care, and even hostile attitudes among the staff. In addition, treatment is usually delivered by relatively inexperienced personnel (Friedman, Quimby, Sufian, Abdul-Quader, & Des Jarlais, 1988).

African Americans have been described as the "second wave" of the AIDS epidemic (Airhihenbuwa, DiClemente, Wingood, & Lowe, 1992). They make up 12 percent of the nation's population but 28 percent of the nation's AIDS patients (Centers for Disease Control, 1991b). But the AIDS epidemic is also striking other ethnic minorities. For example, African Americans and Latinos comprise only 21 percent of the total United States population, yet they account for 43 percent of the AIDS cases reported to the Centers for Disease Control (Centers for Disease Control, 1990). The institutionalized racism that contributes to the increase of the AIDS epidemic among ethnic minorities in correctional facilities is most clearly reflected when the criminal justice system's view of illicit drugs is considered. The national control strategy stresses incarceration as a method to control the supply of illicit drugs and treat drug abuse (Glaser & Greifinger, 1993). On both counts the strategy is failing. The system is failing to incarcerate across color lines (differential sentencing), and those who are incarcerated are not receiving adequate treatment.

Differential Sentencing

Differential sentencing is claimed to be the vent through which America's racism blows (Townsey, 1981). Hinds (quoted in Townsey, 1981) states that "law is the mechanism by which authority implements its intentions." He goes on to describe the prosecution of blacks as an "endless and intricate labyrinth of legal process which holds tantalizing promises of relief but which in practice merely validates the results of proceedings tainted with racism and political expediency." Therefore it becomes extremely clear why blacks in gravely disproportionate numbers experience an unfortunate "confrontation with the criminal law and the selective application of its sanctions" (Townsey, 1981, p. 237).

Clear examples of differential sentencing exist from 1971 surveys in South Carolina. One judge imposed varied sentences in two first-offender marijuana cases. The judge ordered one year's probation and a $400 fine when the case involved a white youth as defendant. The other case involved a black defendant, on whom the judge imposed a two-year sentence (Townsey, 1981).

Even today, differential sentencing for drug possession is having a dramatic effect on the percentage of ethnic minorities in correctional facilities. African Americans and Hispanics are more likely to use crack than cocaine (Dogwood Center, 1995). Even though crack is made by combining cocaine powder with baking soda and heat, a person is likely to receive a harsher sentence if caught with crack. Under the federal guidelines a person caught with five grams of crack (the weight of two pennies) faces a mandatory five-year sentence and a maximum of twenty years (Knight-Ridder, 1994). In contrast, having a similar amount of powder cocaine is a misdemeanor that carries no mandatory minimum sentence and a maximum penalty of one year in jail (Knight-Ridder, 1994). A person would have to possess 500 grams of powder cocaine to receive the same punishment as someone possessing five grams of crack (Knight-Ridder, 1994).

United States District Judge Clyde S. Cahill of Missouri has stated that the federal guidelines for possession of crack have "been directly responsible for incarcerating nearly an entire generation of young Black American men" (Knight-Ridder, 1994). According to the United States Sentencing Commission, during a four-month period in 1992 the racial breakdown of cocaine powder convictions was 45.2 percent white defendants, 29.7 percent black, and 23.3 percent Hispanic. The same time period painted a different picture of crack cocaine convictions: 4.7 percent white defendants, 92.6 percent black, and 2.6 percent Hispanic (Knight-Ridder, 1994). That is a conviction rate ninety times greater for blacks caught with crack than for whites caught with the same drug. Federal statistics from January 20, 1989, to June 30, 1990, revealed that black offenders incarcerated for cocaine offenses during the period had sentences that were 41 percent (on average, twenty-one months) longer than for whites (as cited in Knight-Ridder, 1994).

It appears that in the 1990s, African American drug users have also been targeted for *arrest* nationwide. In 1993, cocaine- and heroin-using blacks were over four times more likely to be arrested for drug possession than cocaine- and heroin-using whites (Dogwood Center, 1995). Fear of arrest for *needle* possesion in black communities targeted for drug-law enforcement discourages black drug users from carrying their own clean needles. This has the unintended consequence of promoting the spread of HIV/AIDS among African Americans (Dogwood Center, 1995).

Injection Drug Users

Due to the national drug control strategy, a growing proportion of injection drug users has emerged in the prison population over the past fifteen to twenty years (Harding, 1995). According to 1991 statistics, nearly one in four state inmates had used a needle to inject illegal drugs during their lives (Harlow, 1993). A history of injection drug use prior to incarceration is present in 95 percent of the cases of AIDS in New York State (Morse et al., 1990). According to Weisbuch (1991), during 1984 and 1985 male-to-male sexual activity was the predominant risk factor associated with contracting the AIDS virus. But by 1988 over half of the new AIDS cases were associated with injection drug use (Weisbuch, 1991).

Since injection drug use is the number one high-risk behavior associated with contracting the AIDS virus among inmates, a logical way to curb the epidemic would be to provide the inmates with the knowledge to protect themselves. Unfortunately, injection drug users are usually blamed for their addiction, rather than offered help.

Lack of Opportunity

Lack of treatment for drug addiction either in or out of the correctional system has a devastating effect on ethnic minorities. Among African American men between the ages of twenty-five and forty-four, AIDS is now the single largest cause of death. Over half of these deaths are drug-related. According to Day (Dogwood Center, 1995), by the end of 1994 over 73,400 African Americans had drug-related AIDS or had died from it. Day also reveals that among persons who inject drugs, African Americans are almost five times as likely as whites to be diagnosed with AIDS. Additionally, almost 80 percent of all new drug-related AIDS cases among African Americans have been reported in the last five years (Dogwood Center, 1995).

The spread of drug-related AIDS also has a devastating effect on Latinos. Almost 28,000 Latinos living in the United States had drug-related AIDS or had died from it by the end of 1994 (Dogwood Center, 1995). Latinos are over three times as likely as whites to be diagnosed with AIDS. Furthermore, of all *new* drug-related AIDS cases among Latinos, over three-quarters have been reported in the last five years.

Hispanic and black populations have a large proportion of men, women, and children with injection-drug-associated AIDS. In the United States, AIDS cases associated with injection drug use in heterosexuals is highest among blacks and Hispanics, 54 percent and 26 percent respectively (Centers for Disease Control, 1988b). In 1994 African Americans had twice the amount of new drug-related AIDS cases (14,400) compared to cases diagnosed in whites (7,200). As Miller, Turner, and Moses (1990) claim, all current research makes it clear that "the burden of AIDS related to IV drug use falls most heavily on minorities."

The necessary treatment for inmates is not growing as fast as the number of prison cells is. The nationwide public policy of mandatory sentencing for drug offenders has led to an increase in prison populations in recent years. For example, the New York State prison population rose from 20,000 in 1979 to 59,000 in 1991, and a large proportion (approximately 82 percent) of the inmates are injection drug users or crack users (Glaser & Greifinger, 1993). The number of drug-related incarcerations in state prisons rose from 8 percent to 26 percent from 1980 to 1994 (Brien & Harlow, 1995). More injection drug users can be found in correctional facilities than in drug treatment centers (Dixon et al., 1993). In 1991, only 1 percent of federal inmates who had moderate-to-severe drug abuse problems had received appropriate treatment (Harlow, 1993).

The AIDS Commission report (1991) states that "meaningful drug treatment" must be made available on demand to convicts both in and out of prison. In addition, the AIDS Commission (1991) cites treatment of chemical dependency as a key factor in improving current conditions in prison and preventing the spread of the AIDS virus as well as future incarceration.

For the few inmates who do complete treatment, there are not enough aftercare programs to help maintain their new lifestyles. Access to follow-up services is an issue needing attention from researchers and policymakers. Post-release relapse is associated with poor housing status, limited social support, lack of drug treatment, and less frequent visits with case managers (Polonsky et al., 1994).

In Maryland's state correctional system, it was found that 50 percent of the inmates diagnosed with HIV infection were potential candidates for anti-retroviral therapy, and 17 percent were severely immune compromised (Kendig et al., 1994). This finding suggests the importance of clinical case management for inmates with HIV infection released to the community in order to establish connections with primary care providers and support services. The prison and community need to work together, since most infected inmates serve short sentences (median three years) (Kendig et al., 1994).

Those who have traditionally held less social power with which to influence the government—blacks and Hispanics especially—have emerged as having the most AIDS cases in prison (Olivero,

1990). Lack of health care prior to incarceration is a barrier for many inmates because they are not only an ethnic minority but part of the drug culture as well (Glaser & Greifinger, 1993). Additionally, inmates who are injection drug users are even less likely than the general population to have received appropriate HIV-directed services prior to incarceration (Dixon et al., 1993). Paradoxically, a period of incarceration may be the only time that many active injection drug users have the opportunity to participate in HIV education and health care programs (Dixon et al., 1993).

Clean Needles

"The need to inject drugs, with no clean needles available" was the most common reason offered by injection drug users for continued needle sharing—despite awareness of inherent AIDS risk (Selwyn, 1987). In one report, 29 percent of the inmates reported using rented or borrowed needles at least half the time or more often (Baxter, 1991). Other items that may retain traces of the IV drug user's blood were also being shared. Approximately half of the inmates shared a cooker (used to heat the drug with water), cotton (used to filter the fluid before drawing it into the syringe), or rinse water (used to clean a syringe after use) with other persons (Baxter, 1991).

It is possible that sterile needles are more accessible and affordable for whites. It has been found that 18 percent of white injection drug users reported using new needles at least half the time, while only 8 percent of African American or Hispanic users reported this behavior (Hutchinson, 1992). Perhaps more troubling, even when selling syringes is legal, some pharmacies will not always sell syringes to African Americans. Evidence from St. Louis confirms that drug stores will not always sell syringes to African Americans even when such sale is legal (Dogwood Center, 1995). Additionally, the police are more likely to confiscate the personal needles of African Americans (Dogwood Center, 1995).

Education

Inequalities in employment, education, and other social institutions appear to deprive minorities of the knowledge and resources needed to protect themselves from AIDS (Hutchinson, 1992). For example, English is the language usually used to inform Spanish-speaking patients that they have AIDS (Hutchinson, 1992). One study has suggested that many Hispanics (especially those who are primarily Spanish-speaking) have received relatively little AIDS education and generally do not perceive themselves to be at risk (Hu, Keller, & Fleming, 1989). Without understanding their afflic- tion, they cannot seek appropriate medical care. Hispanic and African American drug users have reported substantially fewer years of education than their white counterparts (Rogers & Williams, 1987). Less education suggests that Hispanic and African American drug users may be less aware than white drug users of the connection between infection and used or dirty needles (Rogers & Williams, 1987). In the general population, blacks and Latinos have been found to have less knowledge than whites about the facts surrounding HIV and AIDS.

Low Socioeconomic Status

Another factor leading to high-risk behavior among ethnic minori- ties, related to AIDS, is low socioeconomic status. Jerome G. Miller (1995), of the National Center on Institutions and Alternatives, has stated that "[t]he percentage of Americans going in and out of jails is phenomenal. As you go down the socioeconomic ladder, the per- centage gets much higher." In general, inmates are poor, under- educated, and overrepresented by minorities (Glaser & Greifinger, 1993). The Centers for Disease Control and Prevention (1994b) recognizes that "unemployment, poverty, and illiteracy are corre- lated with decreased access to health education, preventive ser- vices, and medical care, resulting in an increased risk for disease. In 1992, 33 percent of Blacks, and 29 percent of Hispanics lived below the federal poverty level, compared with 13 percent of Asians/Pacific Islanders and 10 percent of Whites."

Low socioeconomic status is related to sexual activity and drug use, both high-risk activities associated with contracting the AIDS virus. Lack of economic rewards contributes to early sexual activ- ity (Bowser, 1986). In low-income communities, young people are aware of drug availability and of the harsher elements of society: unemployment, poverty, and racial discrimination. Drug use is a high-risk behavior in relation to contracting AIDS, but it is also an escape from the immediate and harsh reality of the ghettos. The relationship between a lack of adequate social development and the tendency to compensate by using drugs is a salient issue that has been studied by a host of sociologists, psychologists, criminologists, and other researchers.

Lack of Social Marketing

Lack of targeted social marketing to ethnic minority populations has contributed to high-risk behavior. AIDS education endeavors were initially aimed at white gay men. In 1988, a study among fifty-eight county jail inmates—twenty-seven injection drug users and thirty-one noninjection drug users—found that a minority had received formal AIDS education (Valdiserri, Hartl, & Chambliss, 1988). In addition, the messages given were not sensitive to the culture of ethnic minorities and did not reach the African American and Hispanic community (Jimenez, 1987). Many of the social and behavioral programs in ethnic minority communities have failed because they were developed for the dominant group and then implemented into minority communities (Airhihenbuwa, 1989). It has been suggested that the delay in developing culturally sensitive AIDS messages reveals the lack of national interest and concern for the health of minorities (Hutchinson, 1992).

The melting-pot mentality in the United States has led many health professionals to disregard cultural factors. A "salad bowl" concept is alternatively proposed to recognize cultural diversity and the separate and unequal status of different groups in society (Hutchinson, 1992). Within the drug field, ethnic cultures are usually overlooked in favor of the primary culture of drugs (Singer, 1991). AIDS education or treatment must be targeted to a specific group, rather than to all people of color or low-income population, in order to be truly effective (Singer, 1991).

Implications for HIV Programs in Correctional Facilities

Correctional facilities are unique environments. In establishing strategies for conveying information within correctional facilities, policymakers need to consider the content of the message along with who will deliver the message and must not neglect the culture within the facilities.

The Correctional Community as a Subculture

The community must be taken into consideration when developing a health promotion program, and the prison is a community within itself. Strategies for controlling AIDS in correctional facilities should follow closely the strategy for the noninstitutionalized community (Harding, 1987). Persuasive communication and environmental manipulation are two social-influence strategies that have been proposed to encourage health promotion behavior among community populations (Jaccard, Turrisi, & Wan, 1990). Persuasive communication or exposing individuals to information in an attempt to influence and modify individual beliefs, attitudes, and/or decisions has been more readily accepted within correctional facilities. In fact, education is the major intervention to prevent the spread of HIV transmission (Hu, Keller, & Fleming, 1989). Environmental manipulation, a necessary component in behavior change, is lagging in many facilities. Environmental manipulation refers to altering or manipulating structural features in the environment that will provide opportunities for the adoption of health-promoting behavior. In order to control AIDS in prison, inmates should not only be informed about AIDS risk, but they should also be given the opportunity to begin using preventive measures (Harding, 1987).

Neither the means nor the opportunity for safer sex and safe needle practices is available to inmates compared to those living outside prisons. Research suggests that if the means (that is, condoms, needles, and bleach) and opportunity to practice the behavior are available, then a change will take place in sex and drug practices (Baxter, 1991).

In accordance with the theory of harm reduction, strategies that encourage substance users to reduce the harm done by illicit drug use validate the users' competency to protect and help themselves, their loved ones, and their community. Harm reduction accepts drug use as a fact of life and acknowledges its role as a mechanism for coping with the consequences of the social problems previously mentioned, rather than encouraging the "all or nothing" approach to drug use interventions. Essentially, harm reduction encourages starting wherever the person is, and then moving at the pace of the individual. Harm reduction supports individuals in being competent and responsible in their entire lives, including but not limited to their drug using behavior (Harm Reduction Coalition, 1995).

HIV Prevention Message

While some may view needle exchange and access to clean needles as revolutionary, these viable strategies are for reducing HIV transmission. Until policies of correctional facilities change to consider needle exchange, condom distribution, or other protective measures against AIDS, the message from health educators within prisons must reflect the policies of the facility. Even though correctional facilities' administrators recognize the occurrence of high-risk behaviors within the facility, the health program cannot encourage or validate the behaviors. Arguments for behavioral change in correctional facilities by health educators should be applicable to occurrences in the prison and to life on the outside (Baxter, 1991). Possible phrasing, by health educators in correctional facilities, for such arguments include: "things to remember when you are released" and "things to tell your drug using friends during visiting time" (Baxter, 1991).

HIV/AIDS Messengers Within Correctional Facilities

AIDS prevention has also been hindered because of mistrust. Inmates often have mistrust and suspicion when correctional officials express an interest in their well-being. Among inmates, a correlation has been found between rankings of where they got the most information and where they received the most trusted information (Zimmerman, Martin, & Vlahov, 1991). The Department of Corrections was the third-ranked source on both dimensions, with television and newspaper ranked first and second respectively (Zimmerman, Martin, & Vlahov, 1991). A National Health Interview Survey revealed that approximately 85 percent of blacks and Hispanic adults had seen AIDS-related public service announcements on television (Nyamathi & Shin, 1990). Since televisions are not permitted in all correctional facilities, they cannot be the only educational force.

Education by individuals can be most effective when the message is delivered by an individual who shares a cultural and social bond with the target population. An effective AIDS educator is not simply of the same ethnic background, but rather one who is AIDS-literate, comfortable with the target population, and nonjudgmental. Essentially, the message should be given by a spokesperson who is respected by the community (Nyamathi & Shin, 1990). Peer education is the ideal health education/HIV prevention because the diversity of the United States is present in correctional facilities in respect to race, class, gender, and nationality (Berkman, 1995).

Cultural Competency

Much diversity exists among African American and Latino populations, related to culture, values, national origins, and community setting (urban versus rural versus border community) (Nyamathi & Shin, 1990). Culturally competent approaches emphasize a concern for the individual and also incorporate a specific awareness of the cultural and linguistic patterns of the target community. Culturally, Latino and African American women in traditional family roles are responsible for birth control. African American women have been reported to favor contraceptive methods that do not depend on the male partner's behavior (for example, methods other than condoms or withdrawal of the penis). In contrast, Latino women are responsible for birth control, but the authorization of contraceptive use may lie with the husband (Nyamathi & Shin, 1990). Based on this information, AIDS education and condom distribution should be addressed to both partners in the Latino community. Linguistically, direct translation to Spanish does not guarantee an accurate message. Owing to differences in Spanish dialects dependent on national origin (for example, Mexico, Puerto Rico, Cuba), some Latino men did not understand the meaning of the Spanish equivalents of the terms "oral and anal sex" (Peterson & Marin, 1988).

Conclusion

Prison walls effectively restrain criminals, but not the AIDS virus. In 1991, four thousand of New York State's eight thousand inmates who were HIV positive were released (Glaser & Greifinger, 1993). Additionally, because of overcrowding within prisons the "revolving door" phenomenon is common, where inmates appear to be rotated in and out of the correctional system (Polonsky et al., 1994).

The public at large will be protected to the highest degree possible in a system where public health and corrections coordinate their activities toward reducing HIV infection (Weisbuch, 1991). Berkman (1995) asserts that "[t]he chain of common humanity is only as strong as its weakest link, and for the current generation of public health planners, prisons are the breaking point." Historically, the public health profession has been based on social justice. Today, public health professionals must rise to the challenge of advocating for improving inmates' health for the sake of inmates and all of society.

From a public health perspective, the availability of clean needles, condoms, and bleach within correctional institutions would reduce the risk of HIV transmission in those settings (Polonsky et al., 1994). From the correctional point of view, items usable to prevent the spread of AIDS are potential weapons for inmates or could be used to smuggle contraband (Polonsky et al., 1994). The competing ideologies of public health officials and correction officials endanger all of society if the two groups do not coordinate activities. June E. Osborn, chairman of the 1991 National Commission on Acquired Immune Deficiency Syndrome, says: "By concentrating people at highest behavioral risk of HIV, our prisons and jails could be serving as an exceptional place to achieve public health objectives, and especially in the containment of HIV and substance abuse" (AIDS Commission, 1991).

Building more prisons is certainly not the answer to combating AIDS within correctional facilities. On the contrary, less money invested in prisons would allow for society to invest in combatting the social factors delineated in this chapter that contribute to high-risk behavior in relation to HIV/AIDS. As a society, we need to confront the issues analyzed in this chapter that are plaguing the disproportionate number of ethnic minorities in the correctional facilities. When we meet this challenge as a society, we will see a decline in AIDS cases in and out of the correctional facilities.

Chapter Three

An Analysis of Current Educational and Prevention Efforts

The past and current behaviors of social offenders in the prison system increase the risk of HIV infections among incarcerated populations. The rate of HIV infections and AIDS is significantly higher among incarcerated groups than the general population. In fact, correctional institutions have the highest rates of HIV infection of any public institution (Dubler & Sidel, 1989; Morse et al., 1990). Moreover, previously incarcerated social offenders may pose a greater threat of HIV transmission upon release from jail or prison than do other population groups.

Efforts to reduce the incidence of HIV infection among social offenders are complex. They confront numerous policy and program implementation issues for the criminal justice system. Prison officials acknowledge the fact of frequent sexual intercourse within their facilities. But while condom use is the most effective method in preventing HIV infection, the distribution of condoms (considered a contraband) as a strategy to promote safer sex presents a serious dilemma for prison officials.

Another thorny issue that complicates HIV prevention efforts in prison settings is the appropriateness of the intervention. Prison officials are reluctant to provide inmates with information on the avoidance of HIV risk from injection drug use. Although injection drug use is common in prison, inmates do not receive any information on sterilizing hypodermic needles (Vaid as cited in Olivero, 1990). Injection drug use, as well as such behaviors as tattooing, may also increase the risk of HIV transmission in prisons (Carrell & Hart, 1990; Doll, 1988).

The timing of the intervention also presents a logistical problem. Is the appropriate time for program implementation (1) prior to incarceration for those indicted and awaiting due process from the court system, (2) after persons are sentenced and serving time, or (3) upon release from prison during probation or parole or at the completion of the sentence? Furthermore, federal prison system requirements mandate that inmates be tested for HIV prior to release. While some prison facilities test offenders at entry, HIV testing of the incarcerated is voluntary at most correctional facilities.

By March 1993, approximately 8,500 cases of AIDS had been reported in federal and state prison systems, and 3,040 cases were reported by twenty-five city and county jail systems. By 1990, nearly 4.5 million adults were under correctional supervision in the United States, a 75 percent increase since 1983. The number of juveniles in custody also increased significantly from the early 1980s. Also by 1990, more than 760,000 juveniles (590,560 males and 170,084 females) were held in public or private detention facilities (Centers for Disease Control, 1992a). HIV risk behavior may be more prevalent among incarcerated youths, and they may also be less aware of risk-reduction behaviors. African American and other ethnic minority groups are disproportionately incarcerated; as a result, they are disproportionately represented in the prison population.

This chapter identifies current efforts in the published literature on AIDS education and prevention among ethnically diverse prison populations. Furthermore, the chapter provides an analysis of published, quantifiable data on the assessment of HIV seroprevalence, knowledge, and risk behavior in ethnically diverse prison populations.

Basic Approach

This review and meta-analysis seeks to provide background information on any HIV/AIDS educational or prevention activities in the prison setting as well as to guide a formative evaluation process.

The original intent of the literature search was to identify and evaluate the potential effectiveness of new and ongoing HIV/AIDS risk reduction programs in prison settings that target high-risk populations from ethnic minorities. A search of the published literature quickly revealed a dearth of AIDS prevention and intervention programs. Therefore the literature review was expanded to include risk-assessment and risk-reduction studies among ethnically diverse incarcerated populations.

Covering the years 1981 through 1995, an extensive literature search was done using several bibliographic databases: Medline, social sciences, biological sciences, criminal justice, and AIDS. The keys word used in each search included *HIV/AIDS, prisons, seroprevalence, knowledge, attitude, behavior, risk factor,* and *incarceration.* The literature search was restricted to studies in the United States. More than 200 abstracts were initially obtained and reviewed. Ninety-five articles were retrieved, reviewed, and determined to contain the desired, quantifiable data elements. Upon further review, those articles (thirty-two) that specifically stated the racial/ethnic composition of the prison population under study were selected to create the database for the meta-analysis.

Specific data estimates on HIV seropositivity, and on AIDS knowledge, attitude, risk behavior, and self-perceived risk, were extracted from relevant articles, along with racial/ethnic and gender data. While study methods may have varied, the intent of data extraction was to create an analytical database which would include common data items from several studies or items thought to be important for AIDS program planning and evaluation. There was little similarity in methodology or specific outcome measures among the few interventions studies identified. Therefore, each individual education or risk-reduction study was described and the intervention effectiveness critiqued.

The meta-analysis data set contained sixty-five records (or entries). Some articles may have provided data on risk behavior and seroprevalence. Entries were also made for ethnicity-specific or gender-specific data, if such data were provided or could be easily calculated for the published article. Therefore, a single article may have provided data for more than one entry.

Descriptive analytical procedures were used to describe the frequency distribution of study measures; data were summarized by calculating means, and estimate variation was described by the range and standard deviation. The difference between two means was assessed using two-tailed t-test statistics. Simple linear regression analysis was used to describe the relationship between the dependent variable, such as HIV seropositivity, and predictor variables, such as percent ethnic composition of prison population. The slope of the line (Ho: $\beta = 0$) was assessed using F statistics. The strength of the relationship was measured by the coefficient of determination, r^2.

Results of Meta-Analysis

The results of the meta-analysis are presented separately for (1) adult incarcerated populations and (2) adolescent social offenders.

Finding Pertinent to Adults

The HIV seroprevalence rate by ethnic group specified in the study is shown in Table 3.1. "African American" as a percentage of the prison population under study was specified in nineteen entries on HIV seroprevalence. There were thirteen seroprevalence study entries which specified the percentage of Hispanics in the inmate population. There were eleven entries which, in addition to specifying an ethnic group, also grouped persons in a nonspecific "other" category. The twenty entries that described the ethnic population as "nonwhite" were from a single HIV seroprevalence study among men and women from ten federal correctional facilities (Vlahov et al., 1991).

Seroprevalence studies were conducted exclusively among adult inmates. The overall pooled seroprevalence rate estimate for ethnically diverse inmate populations ($n = 43$) was 7.7 percent (range 8–43.4 percent), including one study in which the self-reported seropositivity among women injection drug users was 43.4 percent. In studies in which African Americans comprised a percentage of the prison population, the average seroprevalence rate was 10.7 percent; it was 12.9 percent in studies in which Hispanics were a part of the prison population. In the study that measured HIV seropositivity by ethnicity among incoming offenders, the rate was 5.4 percent among 1,279 African Americans, 8 percent among

Table 3.1. Human Immunodeficiency Virus Seroprevalence Among Ethnically Diverse Incarcerated Adult Populations.

Ethnic Group Specified in Article	n	Range	Mean	Standard Deviation
Pooled Estimate—All Entries	(n = 43)	0.8–43.4	7.7	8.1
African American[a]	(n = 19)	1.0–43.4	10.7	11.1
All African American	(n = 2)	5.4–6.2	5.8	0.6
Hispanic[b]	(n = 13)	1.2–43.4	12.9	12.9
All Hispanic	(n = 2)	0.8–11.6	6.2	7.6
Nonwhite[c]	(n = 20)	2.1–14.7	5.2	3.1
Other[d]	(n = 11)	1.0–25.6	9.6	9.5

[a] Percent African American in inmate population: range = 6.4–79.0 percent (mean = 46.0 percent, standard deviation = 21.7 percent)

[b] Percent Hispanic in inmate population: range = 6.2–37.5 percent (mean = 22.9 percent, standard deviation = 10.7 percent)

[c] Percent nonwhite in inmate population: range = 51.3–93.1 percent (mean = 72.5 percent, standard deviation = 12.7 percent)

[d] Other racial/ethnic groups in inmate population: range = 0.8–22.6 percent (mean = 7.7 percent, standard deviation = 8.3 percent)

243 Hispanics, 9 percent among 2,231 white, and zero among 51 Native American inmates in the Nevada state prison system (Horsburgh, Jarvis, McArther, Ignacio, & Stock, 1990). In the New York prison system, the HIV seroprevalence rate among all African American male inmates was 6.2 percent (2,059); it was 11.6 percent (1,373) among all Hispanic inmates in the same study (LaChance-McCullough et al., 1993).

In regression analysis, HIV seroprevalence rate was not significantly correlated with the African American composition of the inmate population ($r = .12$). The HIV seroprevalence rate was observed to increase, however, as the Hispanic composition of the inmate population increased ($\beta = .712$, $p \sim .001$). In fact, 66 percent of variation in the rate of HIV seropositivity was explained by the percentage of Hispanics in the prison population ($r^2 = .66$). Seroprevalence was also significantly correlated with the other ethnic group composition of the inmate population (r^2 = .59, β = .878, F = 13.13, $p \sim$ .001). There were no statistically significant differences in HIV seropositivity rates among male and female inmates in these analyses. For example, in the study among men and women from the ten federal correction facilities, the mean HIV seroprevalence was 4.1 percent among males and 6.3 percent among females (p = .114).

The ethnic composition of the inmate populations in HIV seroprevalence studies varied significantly. The percentage of African Americans in the adult inmate population ranged from 6.4 percent to 79 percent (m = 46 percent, SD = 21.7 percent). The percentage of Hispanics in the seroprevalence studies inmate population varied from 6.2 percent to 37.5 percent (m = 22.9 percent, SD = 10.7 percent). Few studies included Asians (n = 1) or Native Americans (n = 1). In eleven entries, 1.0–22.6 percent of the ethnic composition of the inmate populations were persons other than African Americans, Asians, Hispanics, or Native Americans. The range of adult inmates specified as nonwhite (n = 20) was 51.3–93.1 percent.

In addition to assessing seroprevalence rates among these ethnically diverse inmate populations, some studies also measured tuberculosis, hepatitis, and syphilis rates (Table 3.2). The rate of tuberculosis in the prison setting ranged from 6.2 percent to 15.1 percent. The rate of hepatitis was 2.3 percent in one of two studies and 67.1 percent in the other. The mean rate of syphilis in inmate populations studied was 14.0 percent, but it varied from 2.0 percent to 35.9 percent. Syphilis seropositivity was correlated with HIV seropositivity (r = .66), although the results were not statistically significant (β = .328, $p \sim$ .05).

Seroincidence studies, which measure the risk of HIV infection in a previously HIV-free population, are relatively rare. Three such studies among ethnically diverse inmate populations were found in the published literature (Horsburgh, Jarvis, McArther, Ignacio, & Stock, 1990; Brewer et al., 1988; Gellert, Maxwell, Higgins, Pendergast, & Wilker, 1993). One study conducted in the Maryland state prison system assayed stored excess sera from male inmates entering between April and June 1985 and April and June 1986. The rate of seroconversion among volunteers (n = 393) later studied in April 1987 was 0.41 percent per inmate-years. The majority of participants were African American (65.2 percent) and relatively young (50.7 percent were under age twenty-five), with 5.7 percent having committed drug offenses and 50.5 percent considered violent offenders. In the Nevada state prison system, the seroincidence rate was 0.19 percent inmate-years among 1,069 inmates who had sera samples obtained at entry (between September and December 1985) and upon release from prison (between August 1987 and July 1988).

The more-than-twofold difference in the seroincidence rate may be due to ethnic composition, other demographic features, and methodological differences between the two studies. Only 48 percent of the inmates in the Maryland state prison study consented to participate. The inmate population in the Nevada state prison study was more ethnically diverse, although the majority of the inmates were white (58 percent). Among ethnically diverse female inmates in an Orange County, California, jail for prostitution, injection drug use, and related offenses, the seroincidence between 1985 and 1991 was 1.6 per 100 inmate-years.

The results of knowledge, attitudes, and behaviors (KAB) surveys among adults are shown in Table 3.3. While the pooled mean percentage of inmates with prior injecting drug use was 31.8 percent ($n = 20$), intravenous drug use among inmate populations was variable (ranging from 3.1 percent to 88 percent among AIDS cases). Injection drug use was not significantly correlated with the ethnic composition of the inmate population. However, injection drug use was strongly correlated with HIV seroprevalence ($r = .79$,

Table 3.2. Seroprevalence of Selected Infectious Diseases Among Ethnically Diverse Incarcerated Adult Populations.

	n	Range	Mean	Standard Deviation
Positive for tuberculosis	($n = 3$)	6.2–15.1	11.7	4.8
Positive for hepatitis	($n = 2$)	2.3–67.2	34.8	45.9
Positive for syphilis	($n = 5$)	2.8–35.9	24.4	13.7
Positive for STD	($n = 1$)	36.5[a]		

a Non-range measure for single study

Table 3.3. HIV/AIDS[a] Knowledge, Attitudes, or Behaviors Among Ethnically Diverse Incarcerated Adult Populations.

	n	Range	Mean	Standard Deviation
Injection drug use	(n = 15)	3.1–53.1	28.6	15.2
Regular condom use	(n = 3)	11.0–45.0	25.0	17.8
Exchange sex for money (F)	(n = 3)	9.8–43.5	24.8	17.2
Sex with bisexual male (F)	(n = 3)	3.0–23.0	9.9	11.3
Sex with person with HIV/AIDS (females)	(n = 1)	0.8[b]		
Sex with male homosexual	(n = 7)	2.8–45.2	14.4	16.6
HIV transmitted via:				
Sexual intercourse	(n = 3)	94.0–96.0	95.0	1.0
Injecting drug use	(n = 3)	94.0–97.0	95.7	1.5
Perinatally	(n = 3)	94.0–96.0	95.3	1.0
Casual contact (F)	(n = 1)	75.0[b]		
AIDS is curable (M)	(n = 1)	91.0[b]		
AIDS is fatal	(n = 3)	96.0–100.0	91.0	2.0
Identify person with AIDS by look (M)	(n = 1)	85.0[b]		
Perceived risk	(n = 4)	45.0–85.0	66.9	20.4
Multiple sex partners	(n = 5)	19.7–47.9	36.8	10.8

[a] Human Immunodeficiency Virus/Acquired Immune Deficiency Syndrome

[b] Non-range measure for single study

F = female, M = male

β = .424, $F_{1,10}$, $p \sim$ .005); injection drug use accounting for 62 percent of the variation in HIV seroprevalence rates (r^2 = .62).

Regular condom use in these analyses ranged from 11 percent to 45 percent; 45 percent of women indicated regular condom use among sex partners. Three studies among women provided data on the exchange of money for sex (Smith et al., 1991; Magura, Kang, Shapiro, & O'Day, 1993; Schilling et al., 1994); 9.8 percent of female inmates in one study, 21 percent in another, and 43.5 percent in the third study reported this prior behavior. About 3 percent of inmates indicated that they had had sex with a bisexual male and 8 percent reported having had sex with a person with AIDS/HIV. Having same-gender sex was reported in 2.8–45.2 percent of adult male inmates.

The knowledge of HIV transmission exceeds 90 percent (Table 3.3). The one exception is casual contact: 75 percent of adult inmates believe that HIV is transmissible by casual contact (such as working with someone with AIDS (Celentano, Brewer, Sonnega, & Vlahov, 1990). One study indicates that 91 percent of inmates believe AIDS is curable; the same study indicates that 85 percent of inmates believe a person with AIDS can be identified by look (Celentano et al., 1990). While self-perceived HIV risk was variable, 45 percent of inmates and 85 percent of incarcerated injection drug users "feared contracting AIDS" (Valdiserri et al., 1988). Inmates having had multiple sex partners ranged from 3.6 percent to 49.6 percent ($m = 36.8$ percent).

Finding Pertinent to Adolescents

Knowledge and risk-behavior factors among adolescents as identified from previous reports are shown in Table 3.4. An average of 11.7 percent of adolescent social offenders in detention centers reported having used intravenous drugs. In the one study which measured condom use, 33 percent of the adolescent detainees indicated having used them regularly. Sex with a bisexual male and sex with a person with AIDS was reported by 1 percent of detainees in each of the two studies identified.

Nearly 90 percent of all adolescent detainees correctly answered survey questions regarding modes of HIV transmission. Also, 87.3 percent of the adolescents believe HIV is transmissible by casual contact, and 64.2 percent of them believe that a person with AIDS can be identified by personal observation. Nineteen percent of incarcerated adolescents in Southern California (Nader, Wexler, Patterson, McKusick, & Coates, 1989) and 69.4 percent of adolescent social offenders in San Francisco (DiClemente, Lanier, Horan, & Lodico, 1991) believed themselves to be at risk of HIV infection. The percentages of adolescents who had multiple sex partners (15–72.9 percent) and multiple lifetime sex partners

Table 3.4. HIV/AIDS Knowledge, Attitudes, or Behaviors Among Ethnically Diverse Incarcerated Adolescent Populations.

	n	Range	Mean	Standard Deviation
Injection drug use	(n = 4)	11.0–12.9	11.7	0.9
Condom use (M)	(n = 1)	33.0[a]		
Sex with bisexual male (M)	(n = 1)	1.0[a]		
Sex with person with HIV/AIDS (M)	(n = 1)	1.0[a]		
Sex with male homosexual	(n = 2)	2.4(M)–13.0(F)	7.7	7.5
HIV transmitted via:				
Sexual intercourse	(n = 2)	89.9(F)–91.8(M)	90.9	1.3
Injection drug use	(n = 4)	85.6–93.6	89.2	4.2
Perinatally	(n = 4)	87.0–90.8	89.0	2.1
Casual contact	(n = 3)	87.0–87.7	87.3	0.4
Identify person with AIDS by look	(n = 1)	64.2[a]		
Perceived risk	(n = 3)	19.0–69.4	49.8	27.0
Multiple sex partners	(n = 2)	15.0–72.9	44.0	40.9
Multiple lifetime partners	(n = 5)	33.3–92.6	73.7	24.0

[a] Non-range measure for single study

(33.3–92.6 percent) reported in the published literature were quite variable. Among youths in the Alabama Department of Youth Services (ADYS), a third (33 percent) were reported to have had more than ten previous sex partners (Lanier & McCarthy, 1989). More than nine in ten (92.6 percent) adolescent offenders in the San Francisco Adolescent Guidance Center reported having two or more lifetime sex partners, whereas 70.9 percent of adolescent offenders in ADYS reported two or more lifetime sex partners (Lanier, DiClemente, & Horan, 1991).

Among adolescents, the average percentage of African Americans among the entries recorded ($n = 8$) was 55.0 percent (range 27.8–74.0 percent); one study was conducted exclusively among African-American male inmates. The average percentage of Hispanics among seroprevalence entries ($n = 6$) was 17.7 percent (range 2.3–50 percent). The range of Asians in the adolescent study population in KAB surveys was 1.4–5.5 percent ($n = 3$).

A study of African American male adolescents awaiting sentencing at a Washington, D.C., area detention center may be particularly noteworthy (Belgrave, Randolph, Carter, & Braithwaite, 1993). In this population of fifty-two detentees, ages 17–22 ($m = 20.6$), AIDS knowledge was reported to be moderate. This adolescent group correctly answered 6 ($m = 5.9$) of 8 items on AIDS knowledge. One-fourth (24.5 percent) believe HIV can be transmitted by mosquitoes, 51 percent by donating blood, and 92 percent believe HIV can be transmitted during sexual intercourse without a condom; 83.7 percent indicated that using condoms can reduce the chances of being infected with HIV. With regard to assessing behavioral intent in this study, 93.8 percent indicated that they would use condoms; 93.8 percent also indicated that they would talk to their partner about safer sexual behavior. More than half (56.3 percent) said they would not engage in sexual activity with more than one person.

Findings Pertinent to Interventions

It appears that the results of interventions to prevent or reduce the risk of HIV disease in the jail or prison setting are only beginning to enter the published literature. The impact of these interventions among select groups, such as injection drug users and parolees, is rather mixed, particularly regarding behavior change (Table 3.5). In a pretest/posttest experimentally designed study among female ($n = 94$) and male ($n = 40$) inmates of a county jail, injection drug users randomly assigned to an eight-hour HIV/AIDS education program over a two-week period did not show any significant change in knowledge or risk behaviors compared to a randomly assigned control group. The majority of 134 volunteer participants

Table 3.5. Select Intervention Studies Among Ethnically Diverse Incarcerated Populations in the United States.

Author/Year/ Location of Study	Study Objectives/Subject	Methods/Description of Intervention	Outcomes Evaluation
Wexler et al. (1994) New York City area, September 1987–December 1990	Evaluate AIDS prevention training program among 394 eligible New York State prison parolees with histories of injection drug use (320 males, 74 females); 57 percent African American, 33 percent Hispanic, 9 percent white, 1 percent others; average age 34.9; paroled within 6 months.	*Adults* Recruited in prison over 20 months March 1988–October 1989, by 10 community-based agencies or by self-referral; eligible with or without prior prison-based drug abuse treatment. 60–90 minute baseline interviews. Intervention included a structured 8-week, 24-session AIDS-focused training program on learning skills, self-help, community therapeutics, and job training. Re-interviewed all program graduates and all eligible who never attended a	Graduates versus comparison groups were less likely to have steady use of intravenous drugs, more likely to always use condoms, and less likely to have had sexual contact with one or more persons who were using injecting drugs, prostituting, or gay or bisexual; no differences in AIDS knowledge, although interaction between program participation and prison-based drug treatment was observed.

Baxter (1991) Maricopa County (Phoenix), Arizona, jail	Evaluate jail-based education and risk assessment program which aimed to decrease risk behavior associated with injecting drug use; 134 volunteers in the Durango jail population, age 35 or younger (82.9 percent), on charges of injection drug use, prostitution, or related activities; 67.2 percent white, 11.2 percent African American, 17.2 percent Hispanic, 4.5 percent Native American.	session at 1 year after base-line interview. Analysis adjusted for variables which differed among graduates and comparison group and were correlated with outcome measures. Pretest/posttest experimental design with random assignment of volunteers to treatment group and control group. Intervention included an 8-hour HIV/AIDS education program over 2-week period, with 6-month post-intervention follow-up.	No significant differences on posttest in change in AIDS knowledge; no statistically significant difference in needle-sharing and sexual behavior although all eleven scales indicated a lower risk for the treatment group at posttest.

Baxter (1991) Maricopa County (Phoenix), Arizona, jail

women ($n = 94$) and men ($n = 40$)

Table 3.5. (continued)

Author/Year/ Location of Study	Study Objectives/Subject	Methods/Description of Intervention	Outcomes Evaluation
Lurigio et al. (1992) Cook County (Chicago), Illinois	Evaluate HIV education program for volunteer adult probationers (n = 99), which aimed to increase HIV knowledge, strengthen risk-reduction behavior intent, and decrease risk behavior; 90 percent male, 86 percent African American, average age 30, average school year completed 11.	Recruited while waiting in lobby of central office of the Cook County Adult Probation Department; random assignment of volunteer to treatment group (HIV education) control days of small group discussion, 14 days for private or one-on-one education; pretest prior to presentation, posttest after presentations, follow-up 12 weeks after education session; 45 percent of HIV-educated and 56 percent of heart disease-educated group participating in follow-up.	HIV-educated group were more knowledgeable than control group on several knowledge items at posttest and at follow-up; no significant difference between HIV education and behavioral intentions at posttest or HIV risk behavior at follow-up.

		Adolescents	
Magura, Kang, Shapiro (1994) New York City Department of Corrections Adolescent Reception and Detention Center, Rikers Island; February 1991–February 1992	Evaluate in-jail voluntary AIDS education curriculum among inner-city adolescents; AIDS education group ($n = 58$) 64 percent African American, 33 percent Hispanic; control group 66 percent African American, 33 percent Hispanic; 16–19 years of age, median 17.8.	Volunteers from 11 dormitories, baseline interview of 411 male inmates, 110 received small-group AIDS education. Follow-up of the first 58 adolescents who received AIDS education upon release from jail; and first 99 who did not follow-up median 10 months after baseline and 5 months after release; 90-minute face-to-face baseline and follow-up interviews. Intervention consisted of four twice-weekly, one-hour small group sessions (8 inmates) which focused on health education issues relevant to drug use and HIV knowledge and risk-reduction behavior.	At follow-up AIDS education participants were significantly more likely than controls to use condoms frequently and had marginally fewer high-risk sex partners; group did not differ by cocaine/crack use or multiple sex partners.

Table 3.5. (continued)

Author/Year/ Location of Study	Study Objectives/Subject	Methods/Description of Intervention	Outcomes Evaluation
Lanier and McCarthy (1989) Alabama Department of Youth Services (ADYS)	Assess the impact of AIDS education on knowledge and attitudes among juvenile offenders at Alabama Department of Youth Services ($n = 415$). Historical data indicated 85 percent males, 56 percent African American, 47 percent age 15 or younger.	Pretest questionnaire to entire ADYS juveniles at entry to and at one institution within ADYS completed 5 days, one-hour/day AIDS instruction several weeks prior to pretest. Instructional program covered basic issues and promoted abstinence as the means of AIDS prevention: youths at a third facility at a group home had not participated in the instructional program. Timing of posttest: no specifics given. Comparison of youths receiving 5 days of instruction to youths who received no instruction.	Reportedly, youths receiving the 5-day instruction were significantly more likely to correctly answer 12 of 14 knowledge items than youths who did not participate in instruction. Participants were more likely to perceive AIDS as a significant problem and themselves at risk as well as tell friends or sex partners if infected.

were white ($n = 134$, 67.2 percent) and under the age of thirty-five ($n = 111$, 82.9 percent), with many admitting to illegal activity ($n = 55$, 41.0 percent) such as prostitution. The ceiling effect—a result of over 80 percent of participants' giving correct responses to thirteen of sixteen knowledge items—may have precluded the detection of any significant change in level of knowledge.

It is noteworthy, however, that all eleven of the scales for needle use and sexual behaviors indicated that the treatment groups had a lower risk of HIV infection than the control group at six-month posttest evaluation (Baxter, 1991), although the results were not statistically significant in this relatively small study sample.

AIDS prevention programs for male ($n = 320$) and female ($n = 74$) parolees with histories of injection drug use did demonstrate significant outcomes differences between those who completed an eight-week, twenty-four-session structured training ($n = 141$) compared to a group who were recruited but never attended the training sessions ($n = 96$). Follow-up interviews after one year of baseline interviews among these New York City area parolees indicate that program graduates were less likely to have injected drugs and were more likely to report safer sex during the follow-up period than the comparison group, after controlling for several covariates in the analyses. Nine percent of graduates with prior prison-based drug treatment and 5 percent of graduates without drug treatment injected drugs steadily during follow-up, compared to 20 percent and 29 percent of persons who never attended a training session, with and without prison-based drug treatment respectively. Among persons with prior prison-based drug treatment, 53 percent of graduates and 4 percent of nonparticipants always used condoms during vaginal intercourse. There was no significant difference between the intervention and comparison group at follow-up with regard to AIDS knowledge, although there were differences between the two groups based on whether study subjects had prior prison-based drug treatment. The majority of the study subjects were African American (57 percent of the total sample), 33 percent Hispanic, 9 percent white, and 1 percent other (Wexler, Magura, Beardsley, & Josepher, 1994).

In an HIV education program for adult parolees of the Cook County (Chicago) jail, those receiving an eighteen-day education session were more knowledgeable about HIV/AIDS at posttest and at follow-up twelve weeks later than was the randomly assigned control group (Lurigio, Petraitis, & Johnson, 1992). While the HIV-educated parolees were more knowledgeable of condom use, type of condom for HIV protection, and blood test for AIDS, the HIV-educated group and control group did not differ with regard to behavior intentions to reduce the risk of HIV infection (that is, cleaning or sharing drug syringes or works, condom use, and talking to sex partners about safer sex).

Studies among adolescent offenders (Table 3.5) indicate that HIV/AIDS education efforts may increase knowledge and change risk perception. Whether HIV risk behaviors can be modified and sustained is yet to be determined. An AIDS education program for incarcerated male adolescent drug users revealed the success of the program for some outcomes measured (Magura, Kang, & Shapiro, 1994). As a result of four twice-weekly small group sessions, the education group ($n = 58$) differed from the control group ($n = 99$) at follow-up (median ten months) in the number of high-risk sexual partners, condom use, and condom acceptability. The education and control groups did not differ, however, on drug use at follow-up.

Among adolescent social offenders at the Alabama Department of Youth Services, youths receiving five-day instructions were more likely than those who did not receive AIDS education (sample sizes not provided) to correctly identify HIV transmission as likely via injection drugs (97 percent versus 88 percent), sexual activity (67 percent versus 57 percent).There were marginal differences between the two groups in perception of self-risk and discussion of HIV/AIDS with sex partners and friends.

Discussion

HIV seroprevalence and risk behaviors are higher among jail and prison inmates than the general population. HIV seroprevalence as well as HIV/AIDS knowledge, attitudes, and behaviors among social offenders are quite variable. Seroprevalence variations are probably related to demographic characteristics (ethnicity and gender), prior risk behaviors, and social offenses (such as illegal drug use and prostitution). While ethnic composition at correctional facilities is also variable, ethnicity in general may be a poor, inconsistent predictor of HIV seroprevalence. The percentage of African

Americans in the inmate population was not correlated with HIV seroprevalence in these meta-analyses. On the other hand, Hispanic ethnicity accounted for 66 percent of the variation in the seroprevalence among inmate populations. Seroprevalence was also strongly correlated ($r^2 = .59$) with ethnicity described in the published literature as "other" (that is, other than white, African American, Asian, Hispanic, and Native American). Such uninformative descriptions of other ethnic groups are useless for HIV/AIDS prevention program planning. In addition to varying by Hispanic ethnicity, injection drug use was also strongly correlated with HIV seroprevalence ($r^2 = .62$); in fact, women injection drug users had the highest HIV seroprevalence reported (43.4 percent). Seroincidence among inmates may be relatively rare (from .19 to .41 per 100 persons). However, among high-risk women injection drug users and prostitutes, it is more common (1.6 per 100 persons).

HIV/AIDS general knowledge is high among adult prison inmates (over 90 percent) and among adolescent offenders (nearly 90 percent). Yet there remain misconceptions of HIV with regard to mosquito, blood testing, and blood donation transmissions (Belgrave et al., 1993). HIV risk behaviors, including sexual activities and drug use, are also variable. Self-perceived risk of HIV infection also appears to be variable and may be related to HIV risk status such as injection drug use and yet undetermined factors.

While most correctional systems provide some form of HIV/AIDS education (Hammett et al., 1994), few carefully designed HIV/AIDS intervention programs are described, or outcome measures evaluated, in the peer-reviewed literature. In general, it is very clear that educational programs are potentially effective in increasing HIV/AIDS knowledge among adult inmates and adolescent social offenders. However, the impact of intervention on changes in risk behavior is yet unknown. Obvious knowledge does not necessarily produce the desired behavior change, and any program effort should have a more comprehensive, theoretically based approach (DiClemente, Lanier, Horan, & Lodico, 1991; Baxter, 1991). While education and risk assessment must be included, prevention efforts that focus on skill acquisition and self-efficacy are most likely to be successful (Belgrave et al., 1993). It is also likely that each HIV educational and prevention program must be individually tailored to suit jurisdictional concerns, correctional system policies, and acceptability to correctional officials (Polonsky et al., 1994). HIV prevention programs must also consider other co-infections in the inmate population, such as tuberculosis, hepatitis, and sexually transmitted disease, which are related to and more common than HIV infections. Since seroincidence in the incarcerated population is rare, intervention should emphasize prior risk behaviors and the reduction of HIV-transmissive behaviors of this selected high-risk population upon release from prisons and jails.

Chapter Four

Prevention and Juvenile Offenders

Few cases of AIDS have yet been reported among confined juveniles, and based on scattered data, HIV seroprevalence rates appear to be very low in juvenile facilities. However, among other evidence, the extremely high rates of STDs among confined juveniles relative to the rates among the corresponding age group in the total U.S. population suggest that many confined juveniles are at risk for HIV/AIDS through unsafe sexual practices, drug use, and other behaviors. This chapter presents findings from the 1994 National Institute of Justice (NIJ)/Centers for Disease Control and Prevention (CDC) survey regarding HIV/AIDS–related policies in juvenile systems. These data reveal that juvenile systems have not as yet mounted the comprehensive, practically oriented prevention programs needed to forestall an incipient HIV epidemic among confined juveniles. The danger is very real and very serious.

The Importance of Comprehensive HIV Prevention Programs

Information alone is not sufficient to induce permanent changes in the often deeply ingrained or addictive behaviors which place adolescents and others at risk for HIV infection. Effective HIV prevention requires approaches that address the complex contexts in which high-risk behaviors occur and persist. However, providing effective HIV prevention programs to confined juveniles is complicated by a central tension: the best programs are explicit about precautionary and preventive measures, yet public opinion and the regulations of juvenile justice agencies often prohibit such explicit messages. Additionally, most systems forbid distribution of materials needed to carry out HIV prevention messages, such as condoms and bleach. While some juvenile justice systems have met this challenge and implemented exemplary HIV education and prevention programs, much work remains to be done in this area. Many juvenile systems currently have only minimal HIV and STD education and prevention programs. Some systems base their lack of programs on very low HIV seropositivity rates among their confined youths. Unfortunately, this argument disregards evidence of substantial levels of high-risk behaviors and STD infection in adolescent populations, particularly those in training schools and detention centers.

Prevention Knowledge Among Adolescents

Research on adolescents' knowledge of HIV and STD transmission has produced mixed results. One study found similarly high levels of knowledge about HIV transmission among confined youths and adolescents in school but also discovered differences in the specificity of knowledge between the two groups and in their motivation to act on that knowledge. Although both confined and in-school youths recognized that sexual intercourse could lead to HIV transmission, confined adolescents were not as motivated to change their behavior, and youths in school were more likely to identify condom use as a way to prevent transmission. These results confirm the need for HIV education programs emphasizing more than the facts of HIV transmission (DiClemente, Lanier, Horan, & Lodico, 1991).

Another study found significant differences in personal efficacy, perceived risk, *and* knowledge between confined and nonconfined adolescents. Given that confined youths are more likely than other adolescents to have lived in poverty, they may simply need better access to health services (Morris et al., 1992). While confined adolescents need basic information on HIV/AIDS, the lack of a sense of personal efficacy and of personal risk is equally troubling.

Types of HIV Education and Prevention Programs

Table 4.1 summarizes the modes of HIV education and prevention employed in juvenile systems. Most systems provide instructor-led education, audiovisual materials, and written materials. However, far fewer systems offer peer education programs.

Instructor-Led Programs

In many juvenile training schools, instructor-led HIV/STD education is offered as part of the health education component of the regular education curricula. The fact that full school programs are offered in these facilities provides an opportunity to reach many confined youths with HIV and STD education. However, the turnover in the population may mean that some, perhaps many, youths do not receive the portion of the curriculum dealing with HIV and STDs.

A particularly well-conceived HIV/STD education program is offered by the Massachusetts Department of Youth Services (DYS)

Table 4.1. HIV/AIDS Education and Prevention for Confined Juveniles.

| | State Juvenile Justice Systems | | City/County Detention Centers | |
| | (n = 41) | | (n = 32) | |
	n	percent	n	percent
Instructor-led education[a,b]	38	93%	27	84%
Peer education programs[b]	10	24	5	16
Audiovisuals[b]	35	85	25	78
Written materials[b]	37	90	25	78

a Instructor-led education involves the participation of a trained leader in some substantial part of a session.

b Programs provided in at least one facility in the system.

Source: NIJ/CDC questionnaire responses, 1994.

Two full-time educators funded through CDC's HIV prevention cooperative agreement with the state's Department of Public Health cover HIV and STD issues in the context of a comprehensive sexuality education program. DYS educators take an extremely positive, respectful approach to the youths that is sensitive to their diverse learning levels, emotional states, and cultural backgrounds. Rather than lecturing, preaching, or patronizing them, the presenters have developed a highly innovative, interactive approach. While this is, strictly speaking, instructor-led education, it is also really youth-centered. The educators spend significant time bonding with the youths and listening to their concerns. They seem able to develop trusting relationships with the youths even in the context of one-time sessions in detention facilities.

In longer-term facilities, the DYS educators offer a series of four ninety-minute sessions. During the first session at these facilities, the educators ask the youths to select the particular topics and issues they would like to cover during the series. The youths discuss the issues and vote on those they would like to address in class. This approach shows respect for their feelings and concerns but is also flexible enough for the educators to integrate their agenda with that of the youths and cover the important points they have prepared. The educators also create exercises and materials addressing the particular topics the youths have chosen.

Another important part of the DYS four-session series is a visit from an HIV-infected guest. Unlike most such programs, the guest does not simply tell his or her story, drawing appropriate lessons about risk behaviors; rather, he or she is interviewed by the youths. They are permitted to ask any questions they want, as long as they are respectful of the guest. They generally ask appropriate questions and the guest responds with useful information they can apply to their own lives in practical ways.

Finally, the Massachusetts program places a heavy emphasis on education for staff. By conducting sessions with staff, the educators build support for their program and help the other staff understand its importance to the youths. Moreover, a staff that is better educated on HIV and sexuality issues is better equipped to provide information and follow up in the facility during the majority of hours when the HIV educators are not present.

Peer-Led Programs

Several juvenile systems and facilities have implemented HIV peer education programs. In New Mexico, HIV prevention education is part of a peer drug and alcohol prevention education program, started seven years ago as part of the Drug-Free Schools Program Approximately twenty confined juveniles act as peer educators each year. In one session of this series, confined juveniles learn how HIV is transmitted and how to practice safer sex, discuss their fears of HIV, and receive referrals for HIV testing (D. Martinez, New Mexico Department of Children, Youth, and Families, personal communication, May 12, 1995).

In Los Angeles County, the Peer HIV Education Research Project (PHERP) was designed to compare the effectiveness of peer and adult educators. Peer educators team-teach classes with adult teachers, covering prevention and transmission of HIV including safer sex and injection practices, alcohol and drug abuse, STD symptoms and treatment, and negotiation skills regarding condom use. Students participate in role playing exercises and listen to an HIV-positive guest speaker discuss issues of living with HIV disease. At the beginning and end of the program, participants are surveyed on their HIV knowledge (J. Anderson, Peer HIV Education Research Project, May 12 and 16, 1995). The program also surveyed half of the juveniles three months after the intervention, at which point at least some of the participants had returned to the community. Initial evaluation results show that each type of educator has different strengths. Although differences were quite small, peer-led groups showed more positive changes in attitude and behavior, while adult-led groups demonstrated higher levels of HIV knowledge (staff of Peer HIV Education Research Project, personal communication, February 2, 1996).

Written Materials

Effective HIV prevention education must employ materials appropriate to the reading abilities and cultures of confined juveniles. Juvenile systems reported using HIV education materials with an average sixth-grade reading level. However, four jurisdictions reported using materials with reading levels of tenth to twelfth grade, and one reported using materials with a third-grade reading level. It appears that the reading level of materials is appropriate in most responding systems.

Communities of color are overrepresented in confined populations and among adolescents with AIDS. Therefore, culturally specific HIV prevention materials should be available in training schools and detention centers. Similarly, confined juveniles whose first language is not English should have access to HIV prevention materials in a language in which they are fluent. Materials addressing issues facing females specifically should also be available. Although some juvenile systems provide multicultural HIV and STD prevention materials, too many continue to provide general information only.

Topics Covered in HIV and STD Education

Discussing sex with young people is complicated and controversial. The CDC has encouraged input from parents and community in forming HIV prevention curricula for public schools (Centers for Disease Control, 1988a). Obtaining meaningful community input into education for confined juveniles may be more difficult. However, because all methods of HIV prevention depend on individual behavior, frank and honest discussion of how HIV is transmitted is essential.

All but one state juvenile system, and most city/county systems, responding to the NIJ/CDC survey reported covering basic HIV and STD information in their education programs. However, it appears that many more state systems than city/county systems cover topics such as safer sex, the meaning of tests for HIV or STDs, negotiating skills, condom use, self-perception of risk, and others of importance. The fact that juveniles remain in city/county detention centers for much less time than in state training schools, reducing the opportunity to provide extensive HIV and STD education, may explain some of this discrepancy. However, in light of the research literature, topics such as self-perception of risk and efficacy of prevention activities are particularly important.

Condom Distribution

Many adolescents engage in sexual activities that put them at risk for HIV infection. Only two jurisdictions (Alameda and San Mateo, California) reported making condoms available to confined juveniles for use within the facility, and only one additional jurisdiction (Miami) reported plans to distribute condoms in the future. However, 40 percent of state systems and 32 percent of city/county systems reported that they make condoms available to juveniles when released.

HIV Testing Policies

Only two state juvenile systems (5 percent), Mississippi and New Mexico, and no city/county detention centers reported mandatory HIV antibody testing of incoming juveniles. The vast majority of state juvenile systems (95 percent) and city/county detention centers (84 percent) provide voluntary testing and/or test for HIV when juveniles show symptoms of HIV disease (83 percent of state systems and 88 percent of city/county detention centers). This policy decision may be due in part to the high cost of mass screening programs or the perceived low rates of infection among confined juveniles. Although early detection might permit early medical intervention for HIV-infected juveniles, most systems have found it preferable to provide testing services on a voluntary basis combined with education programs.

Eight state juvenile systems (19 percent) and three city/county detention centers (9 percent) reported conducting mandatory testing of pregnant girls. This will be an important policy to monitor, in view of recent evidence that treatment of HIV-positive pregnant women with zidovudine (ZDV) reduces the risk of perinatal transmission.

Although it is often assumed that those who are at elevated risk and/or are HIV infected will volunteer for HIV testing, many high-risk individuals may not come forward to be tested out of fear of the results (Behrendt et al., 1994). However, early treatment including prophylaxis for *Pneumocystis carinii pneumonia* (PCP) or other opportunistic infections, immunizations, and counseling regarding diet and food preparation to avoid food-borne pathogens may lengthen and improve the quality of life for HIV infected juveniles.

In addition, voluntary HIV testing for juveniles may be complicated by parental-consent requirements. Having to acknowledge high-risk behavior to their parents may discourage juveniles from pursuing voluntary testing. Thirty-seven state systems (90 percent) and twenty-five city/county detention centers (78 percent) reported that juveniles do not need parental consent in order to be tested for HIV infection. However, only five states (California, Colorado, Iowa, Michigan, and Washington) explicitly allow minors to consent to HIV testing (Morris et al., 1992). In implementing successful voluntary HIV testing programs, juvenile justice systems administrators must consider how to make testing accessible in addition to providing confidential services, extensive education, and quality medical care.

Confidentiality and Disclosure

Ensuring confidentiality of HIV test results is one of the most important ways to encourage youths to be tested. In juvenile justice systems this can be both very complicated and very difficult. Although few juvenile justice systems officially follow a policy of disclosure to nonmedical staff, this disclosure can be difficult to prevent in practice. Further, although by official policy only 25 percent of systems notify parents or guardians of their children's HIV status, often parents have general access to their children's medical records. Parents have good reasons for wanting to know the HIV status of their children, particularly if their children are at high risk for HIV infection. However, adolescents may also have valid concerns about informing their parents of their HIV status. Juvenile justice systems should carefully consider all ramifications before informing parents or guardians of HIV status without the consent of the juvenile. Indeed, in many jurisdictions such disclosure without consent may be illegal.

Almost all systems reported a policy of notifying the juvenile (96 percent), her or his doctor (85 percent), and the local public health department (80 percent) of HIV status. At least half of the systems also reported policies for notifying other medical staff (63 percent), institution management (50 percent), and spouses or sexual partners of HIV infected youths (49 percent). A partner-notification policy might mean that the confined juvenile notifies the partners directly, that juvenile justice staff notify the partners, or that public health authorities are notified and follow up with the partners. Only 20 percent of responding systems reported a policy of notifying nonmedical juvenile justice staff.

HIV Pretest and Posttest Counseling

Pretest and posttest counseling are critical components of programs dealing with HIV in juvenile justice systems. More than half (59 percent) of state systems and 22 percent of city/county detention centers reported providing HIV prevention counseling in some or all of their facilities. Overall, approximately two thirds of all facilities in the systems responding to the NIJ/CDC survey reported providing HIV prevention counseling.

In order to maintain confidentiality, posttest counseling must be individual. Individual pretest counseling can encourage youths to express their feelings honestly and benefits them with increased individual attention. However, limited resources often preclude offering this service. Sixty-two percent of state systems and 38 percent of city/county systems reported providing individual HIV prevention counseling. More than half of the participating state juvenile justice systems reported providing HIV prevention counseling covering the meaning of HIV antibody test results, safer sex practices, condom use, effects of alcohol and drug use on HIV risk, self-perception of risk, and/or referrals to other services.

STD Testing and Notification

Many more systems perform routine screening for syphilis, gonorrhea, and chlamydia than perform screening for HIV. STD testing on request and in cases of clinical indications is reportedly available in the vast majority of juvenile justice systems. Similarly, more systems require that sexual partners be notified of juvenile syphilis, gonorrhea, and chlamydia infection than HIV infection. Approximately 80 percent of participating systems reported having policies requiring sexual partner notification of syphilis and gonorrhea infection, and 75 percent of systems reported having a policy requiring sexual partner notification of chlamydia infection. However, as with HIV notification policies, very few systems (5 percent of state systems, 13 percent of city/county detention centers) officially require notification of parents or guardians when a confined juvenile tests positive for an STD.

Pregnancy Testing

Sixty-four percent of state juvenile justice systems reported policies for routine pregnancy testing. This is more than three times the proportion of city/county detention centers that reported such policies (19 percent). The difference is likely due to the short length of stay in juvenile detention centers. However, almost all systems (94 percent), both state and local, reported testing girls who demonstrate symptoms of pregnancy, and almost all systems (94 percent) reported providing voluntary pregnancy testing. Pregnancy testing of HIV-positive girls may become increasingly important in light of research findings suggesting the efficacy of early intervention with ZDV in preventing perinatal transmission of HIV.

Conclusion

Because many juveniles in confinement have engaged in activities in the community that place them at elevated risk for HIV and other STDs, and because HIV has not yet become as widespread as other STDs among adolescents in detention centers and training schools, a unique opportunity for HIV prevention currently exists. Some juvenile systems have implemented impressive programs, but much work remains to be done. If juvenile justice systems do not seize this opportunity, HIV infection among confined juveniles will likely escalate.

Chapter Five

Policy Response to a Public Health Opportunity

HIV/AIDS is a serious problem in many correctional systems, as demonstrated by the statistics presented in Chapter One. But as was also suggested earlier, there is an important public health opportunity to respond effectively to HIV/AIDS in correctional populations because they represent perhaps the highest concentrations found anywhere in the United States of persons already infected with HIV and those at high risk through drug use and sexual contact. As literally "captive audiences," inmates are thus at least logistically easier to reach with education, prevention, and treatment programs. Have correctional systems taken full advantage yet of this public health opportunity? The answer is decidedly no, although some systems have done much better than others. By and large, however, inmates remain quite seriously underserved.

Guidelines promulgated in 1993 by the World Health Organization's Global Programme on AIDS call for programs of education, prevention, and treatment to apply "equally to prisoners and the general community. . . . [N]on-discriminatory and humane care" of inmates with HIV disease, according to the WHO guidelines, means no mandatory testing, segregation, or programmatic restrictions based on HIV status. Rather, on-request testing, comprehensive prevention programs "based on risk behaviors actually occurring in prisons," and "health care equivalent to that in the community" should be provided (World Health Organization, 1993).

In the view of many, correctional systems in the United States have fallen far short of adhering to these standards in their policy response to HIV/AIDS. The National Commission on AIDS, for example, released a report which was sharply critical of the correctional response in virtually all policy areas. The Commission stated that "[t]he situation today for many prisoners living with HIV disease is nothing if not 'cruel and unusual'. . . . [T]oo many correctional facilities subject inmates to a series of unnecessary, arbitrary indignities which fundamentally affect their basic human rights." Medical care, psychosocial services, drug treatment, education and prevention programs, counseling and testing services, confidentiality and notification procedures, and programs specifically targeting women are all seriously deficient in correctional facilities, according to the Commission's report. The Commission recommended that the U.S. Public Health Service take the lead in developing and promulgating guidelines for prevention and treatment of HIV disease in prisons and jails (National Commission on AIDS, 1991). While the Centers for Disease Control and Prevention (CDC) have issued detailed guidelines for the prevention and control of tuberculosis in correctional facilities, no such guidelines have yet been issued for HIV/AIDS. In the mid-1980s, CDC attempted to achieve consensus on guidelines for correctional facilities but was unable to do so.

Thus the ineffectiveness of correctional systems' policy responses to the HIV/AIDS epidemic represents not only a missed public health opportunity but also a failure in ethics and human rights. However, the correctional systems themselves should not bear sole responsibility for this failure. There has been a notable neglect of prisons and jails by public health agencies and by community-based organizations. Because prisoners have little political influence and the public is mainly interested in keeping them locked up, there is really no one to speak for them and their interests. Efforts to foster dialogue among, and mutual understanding of, the differing but not necessarily opposing perspectives of correctional officials, public health officials, and community groups hold promise for more cooperative and ultimately more effective responses to HIV/AIDS in prisons and jails. Such dialogue has been undertaken in Canada and has helped encourage the view that "the promotion of health in prisons does not necessarily entail lessening of the safety and security of prisons. . . . Indeed, promotion of health in the prison population and the education of both prisoners and staff may be the best ways to create safety and security" (Jurgens, 1994a). Thus there may be common ground on which to build. Clearly, in any case, developing and implementing policy on HIV/AIDS in prisons and jails is a complex and challenging enterprise for all concerned. This chapter details efforts in the following areas:

- Education and behavioral interventions
- Precautionary and preventive measures
- Testing, counseling, confidentiality and disclosure
- Housing and correctional management
- Medical care and psychosocial services
- Discharge planning and post-release services

Much of the data presented in this chapter comes from the 1994 NIJ/CDC survey of prison and jail systems.

HIV and STD Education and Behavioral Interventions

Education and prevention programs probably represent the most important policy response to HIV/AIDS in correctional settings. This section characterizes ideal and existing programs.

The Importance of Comprehensive Correctional HIV/STD Prevention Programs

Prisons and jails are important settings for HIV/STD education and prevention efforts, because of the high concentrations among inmates of persons already infected with HIV and those with histories of injection and other drug use, high-risk sexual practices, and other behaviors that may place them at elevated risk for infection. In addition, inmate populations are literally captive audiences, available for education and intervention programs for the length of their stays in correctional facilities. Moreover, virtually all prisoners return to the community, so helping them to reduce their risk-taking behavior benefits not only them but also others they may encounter in the outside world. Finally, high recidivism rates mean that substantial populations of infected and at-risk persons are continuously cycling in and out of correctional facilities, further fueling the epidemic within and outside the walls.

The importance of seizing the opportunity to implement comprehensive, high-quality HIV/STD education and prevention programs in prisons and jails is, or should be, well known. To date, however, correctional systems have largely missed this opportunity. Moreover, few individuals being released from prisons and jails are able to access long-term support systems in the community to help them make and sustain difficult behavioral changes.

An abundance of research makes clear that information alone is insufficient to induce permanent changes in the often deeply ingrained or addictive behaviors that place people at risk for HIV infection. Instead, effective HIV prevention requires comprehensive approaches that address the complex contexts in which high-risk behaviors occur and persist. A recent report of the Institute of Medicine calls for integration of individual concepts such as "self-efficacy" (that is, the individual's belief in his or her ability to act in a certain way) with sensitivity to how broader gender and socio-cultural factors influence individual behavior choices (Auerbach et al., 1994). Those factors include the values and historical experiences of variously defined groups: couples, social networks, cultural and other communities, the society as a whole.

Drawing on their perception that the epidemiology of HIV/AIDS in the United States represents "multiple localized epidemics," three leading researchers have recently called for a two-level prevention program composed of universal and targeted elements. The universal components should include dissemination of basic information on HIV/AIDS and risk-reduction methods, efforts to reduce discrimination based on HIV status, and removal of restrictions on access to condoms, sterile needles, and other materials needed to implement guidelines for safer behavior. In addition, communities with high prevalence and/or risk of HIV/AIDS (surely including correctional facilities, although they are not specifically enumerated by the authors) should be targeted with intensive interventions. These interventions should address the "physiologic, emotional, interpersonal and cultural contexts" of behavior and emphasize the following strategies: "communicating face to face in understandable language . . . changing peers' attitudes toward sex and drug use, teaching new technical and social skills . . . , providing the means for safer behavior . . . [and continuously assisting persons] to avoid relapses into unsafe behavior" (Des Jarlais, Padian, & Winkelstein, 1994; Rogers & Osborn, 1993).

Correctional HIV prevention efforts have thus far emphasized education or provision of information. The other necessary elements of a comprehensive HIV prevention program have been largely missing. Too little attention has been paid to the very serious social, cultural, economic, and psychological barriers to HIV-related behavior change (Correctional Association of New York AIDS in Prison Project, 1994). Harm-reduction and risk-reduction strategies have been insufficiently addressed in correctional HIV education programs, often because authorities are reluctant to teach about proscribed behaviors, such as sex and drug use, and to provide the means to render these activities safer.

The challenge of providing effective HIV education and prevention for correctional inmates is thus heightened by a central tension: the best programs seem to be those that are most explicit about particular precautionary and preventive measures, yet correctional regulations often prohibit such explicit messages and, in any case, almost universally prohibit the distribution of condoms, bleach, and other materials needed to implement them.

The State of Knowledge Among Inmates

Knowledge is a first step in HIV prevention. However, in correctional facilities, as in the world outside, simply knowing what behaviors place one at risk for HIV usually does not translate into avoidance of these behaviors. There also continues to be discrimination against HIV-infected persons, possibly based on misinformation or occurring in spite of generally accurate understanding of transmission factors. A survey of Virginia inmates, for example, revealed that most were reluctant to be around persons with HIV even though they had a good understanding of how the virus is transmitted (Ibrahim, 1994).

Inmates are probably better informed about HIV now than they were in the middle and late 1980s, when irrational fear about AIDS, sometimes approaching hysteria, gripped many correctional facilities. A number of surveys document that most inmates and correctional staff understand the major means of HIV transmission. Still, areas of uncertainty and misinformation remain. In the Virginia survey cited above, most respondents knew that HIV is transmitted through sex and needle use, but many were uncertain how transmission actually occurred during these activities. Almost one-fourth of both male and female inmates in Virginia thought HIV could be transmitted only during same-gender sexual contact but not during heterosexual contact. At the same time, over 90 percent of both males and females said it was unsafe to have a blood transfusion, nearly half thought HIV could be transmitted through saliva, and one-fourth believed transmission could occur through sharing dishes or utensils. Misinformation about transmission through other forms of casual contact also persists among Virginia inmates (Ibrahim, 1994). Only about half of Oregon inmates attending HIV education workshops gave correct answers to pretest questions regarding the body fluids through which HIV may be transmitted, the most risky practices for HIV transmission, and the length of the "window period" between infection and development of detectable antibodies (Oregon AIDS Support [Inmate] Services, 1994).

Another issue that must be taken seriously in the planning and execution of HIV education programs is the extent to which certain groups, especially blacks, believe that HIV was deliberately introduced for genocidal purposes. This belief is apparently widespread among black inmates in New York State and elsewhere (D. Gilbert, inmate, personal communication, November 10, 1994). This makes it even more important to have HIV education and prevention programs offered by persons with credibility among inmates, and to institute peer-based programs.

Types of HIV Education and Prevention Programs

Table 5.1 summarizes the types of HIV education and prevention programs provided by correctional systems according to the 1994 NIJ/CDC survey. It suggests a troubling emergent pattern: the continuing decline from 1990 to 1994 in the percentage of state and federal prison systems that provide instructor-led HIV education for inmates, that is, face-to-face educational sessions led by trained instructors at which inmates have the opportunity to ask questions. In 1994, 75 percent of prison systems reported providing instructor-

Table 5.1. HIV/AIDS Education and Prevention for Inmates, November 1992 to March 1993/1994.

| | U.S. State/Federal Prison Systems | | | | U.S. City/County Jail Systems | | | |
| | November 1992 - March 1993 (n = 51) | | 1994 (n = 51) | | November 1992 - March 1993 (n = 31) | | 1994 (n = 29) | |
	n	%	n	%	n	%	n	%
Instructor-led education[a,b]	44	86	38	75	18	58	18	62
Peer education programs[b]	17	33	18	35	3	10	2	7
Videos/ audiovisual[b]	49	96	45	88	28	90	19	66
Written materials[b]	49	96	48	94	22	71	21	72

[a] Instructor-led education involves the participation of a trained leader in some substantial part of a session.

[b] Programs provided in at least one facility in the reporting correctional system.

Source: NIJ/CDC questionnaire responses.

led education in any of their facilities. Sixty-two percent of city and county jail systems, about the same as in 1992, reported instructor-led inmate education in 1994.

Peer-based HIV education programs were reportedly offered in 35 percent of state and federal prison systems and in only 7 percent of city and county jail systems. The small percentage of jail systems offering peer programs is no doubt partially explained by the high turnover and short average length of stay in these facilities. There has been little change in these percentages since 1992.

Audiovisual and written materials on HIV/AIDS are used in the majority of systems, but the percentages of systems reporting their use has declined since 1992.

The reasons for the continuing decline in attention to HIV/AIDS education and prevention in correctional facilities are unclear. But they may include dissipation of the earlier crisis atmosphere regarding AIDS, lack of attention to HIV issues in the outside community surrounding the facilities, and resource constraints. In any case, the trend is troubling. Correctional facilities are key loci for ongoing HIV prevention work, but clearly many systems are not taking full advantage of this opportunity.

The 1994 NIJ/CDC survey provides further evidence of missed opportunities to provide HIV/AIDS prevention and education programs for inmates. Less than one-third (29 percent) of state and federal prison systems provided instructor-led HIV education in all of their facilities, and 12 percent did not know how many facilities provided such programs. Only one state prison system reported offering HIV peer education in all of its facilities. Almost half of the state and federal systems reported that HIV prevention counseling was offered and audiovisual materials on HIV/AIDS were used in all their facilities, while almost two-thirds said written materials on HIV/AIDS were distributed in all their institutions.

The above findings are based on the responses of correctional systems' central offices regarding coverage of their facilities by different HIV education and prevention methods. Over the years since the NIJ/CDC survey series began, there have been concerns raised about the accuracy of information provided by systems' central offices. Therefore, in 1994 abbreviated questionnaires focusing on policies were sent to samples of individual facilities in selected state and federal correctional systems so that their responses could be compared with those submitted by central offices.

Validation study results for aspects of HIV education and prevention programs reveal varying levels of agreement between central office and facility responses. For example, in three systems whose central offices reported that all of their facilities provided instructor-led HIV education, in fact 80 percent of the individual facilities reported that they offered instructor-led education. There were analogous rates of agreement for HIV prevention counseling (100 percent), use of audiovisuals (87 percent), and distribution of written materials (91 percent). Further discussion of each of the major methods of HIV education and programming is provided below.

Instructor-Led Education. Instructor-led education is a basic means of providing information on HIV/AIDS, risk factors for HIV transmission, and methods of reducing inmates' risk of acquiring and transmitting HIV. Intake and ongoing education and prevention programs offer the chance to educate inmates about the particular risks they may encounter in a correctional facility and help them reduce their high-risk behaviors, while prerelease programs afford an important opportunity to reinforce risk-reduction messages and strategies as individuals are returning to the community.

In addition to the extent to which facilities within a system are actually offering particular education programs, it is important to know the extent to which inmates in facilities providing such programs are actually attending them. An indication is provided by learning whether attendance is mandatory. Seventy-one percent of state/federal systems report that HIV education sessions are mandatory for all incoming inmates, while 24 percent report mandatory sessions for current inmates and 25 percent for inmates about to be released. Validation study results suggest that over half of the facilities in systems with policies that HIV education be mandatory for inmates about to be released are not abiding by these policies.

Table 5.2 shows the topics that correctional systems report as covered in their HIV/AIDS education programs. This indicates that topics such as basic HIV information, alcohol and drug risks, and safer sex practices are widely covered. However, smaller percentages of systems include practical prevention skills such as proper condom use, safer injection practices, and pregnancy choices. These topics may be more controversial (for instance, pregnancy termination) or difficult to address because the means to implement the messages (condoms, bleach, sterile injection material) are largely prohibited to inmates as a matter of correctional policy and/or law. In addition, fewer systems include topics such as negotiation skills for safer sex, identifying barriers to behavioral change, triggers for relapse, and coping skills that are best covered in ongoing prevention programs rather than in "AIDS

Table 5.2. Topics Covered in HIV/AIDS Education
for Inmates, 1994.

Topics	U.S. State/Federal Prison Systems (n = 51)		U.S. City/County Jail Systems (n = 29)	
	n	%	n	%
Basic HIV information	48	94	23	79
Meaning of HIV test results	43	84	22	76
Safer sex practices	44	86	22	76
Negotiation skills for safer sex	20	39	17	59
Proper condom use	30	59	19	66
Safer injection practices	28	55	16	55
Tattooing risks	45	88	17	59
Alcohol/drug risks	46	90	22	76
Self-perception of risk	32	63	18	62
Identifying barriers to behavioral change	28	55	19	66
Triggers for behavior relapse	19	37	18	62
Coping skills	24	47	15	52
Referral to other services	37	73	18	62
Vertical transmission of HIV	40	78	19	66
Pregnancy choices	29	57	14	48

Source: NIJ/CDC questionnaire responses.

101" or similar introductory education sessions. Indeed, these lower percentages suggest that few systems are actually providing ongoing HIV prevention programs.

Validation study results on topics that according to central office responses are supposed to be covered in HIV education suggest some interesting patterns. In general, the percentages of facilities in agreement on topic coverage are higher than the percentages of agreement regarding topics not supposed to be covered. For example, in twelve systems where safer sex practices were supposed to be covered in HIV education, 88 percent of the facilities in the validation study reported that this topic was indeed included. On the other hand, in five systems where safer injection practices were not supposed to be covered in HIV education, two-thirds of the facilities reported covering this topic anyway. Thus, at least some individual facilities seem inclined and able to expand their educational programs beyond the topics specified or authorized by their systems' central offices. This should not be completely surprising since, in most systems, wardens, superintendents, and health services staff retain substantial influence over how programs and policies are implemented in individual facilities. Thus, at least some facilities appear able to circumvent the limits placed by systems on the content of HIV education and prevention programs.

One of the key features of a targeted HIV prevention program is "communicating in understandable language." Since many inmates are not native English speakers, this should include offering education in non-English languages. Survey responses indicate that only 39 percent of state/federal prison systems and 41 percent of city/county jail systems provide HIV education in Spanish.

Beyond simple linguistic understandability, there is the question of credibility. In general, there is likely to be substantial inmate mistrust of information provided by correctional staff, particularly on controversial topics such as HIV/AIDS. Therefore, correctional systems should seriously consider having inmate peers or outside groups, such as public health departments or AIDS service organizations, provide HIV education in their facilities. Many such organizations are ready and willing to provide services, and their utilization can help correctional systems make significant budget savings.

Survey results indicate that correctional systems are already making fairly widespread use of outside resources for HIV education. While 98 percent of state/federal prison systems use their own medical staffs to provide HIV education, 80 percent also report using public health departments, 56 percent report using AIDS service organizations, and 31 percent say they use inmate peer educators. Among responding city/county jail systems, two-thirds report relying on their own medical staffs. But two-thirds also report using public health departments, 52 percent use AIDS service organizations, and only 10 percent report use of inmate peer educators.

The practical implementation of programs that look good on paper may pose problems. For example, New York State mounted an apparently ambitious public health department-based HIV education effort for inmates. In 1990, the state health department's AIDS Institute was funded to provide basic HIV education sessions for inmates and staff, as well as testing and counseling services to the entire state prison system (LaChance-McCullough et al., 1993, 1994). An inmate who has been active in efforts to establish inmate peer education programs on HIV in New York stated that the AIDS Institute's "Criminal Justice Initiative" resulted in some improvements in programs, including having more sessions presented by people with street experience in a language and style more understandable to inmates, and the availability of anonymous HIV testing. However, the inmate asserted that some of the promised improvements were not carried out or sustained. The peer education programs supposed to be set up by the AIDS Institute did not materialize (anonymous inmate, personal communication, November 10, 1994). An assessment based on focus groups with inmates in New York City jails and former New York State prisoners found a range of experience with HIV educational programs in correctional facilities. Generally, women reported more exposure to HIV education while incarcerated. By contrast, some men said they had been in facilities with no HIV education or prevention programs (Mahon, 1994b).

In the Oregon state prison system, HIV education and pretest/posttest counseling has been provided since 1987 by Correctional Treatment Services (CTS), which is staffed and housed by the State's Mental Health Division but funded by the Department of Corrections. This arrangement has generally worked well to dissociate the provision of education and counseling from the correctional system. CTS educators and counselors appear to have developed excellent credibility with both inmates and correctional staff. The authors observed HIV education sessions at men's and women's facilities in Oregon. The CTS educator was extremely knowledgeable and effective in developing rapport with the inmates. She spoke in frank and understandable terms of situations and issues that were relevant to the experiences of this population, encouraged and elicited substantial inmate participation, and offered clear, practical guidelines for risk reduction (C. Schroeder, L. Fanning, & others at Correctional Treatment Services, personal communications, September 19–20, 1994).

Achieving consistency of program quality, topic coverage, and factual information provided in HIV education become particularly complex and challenging issues in large correctional systems with multiple facilities. An innovative approach has been taken by the Florida system, which employs video teleconferencing to present simultaneous HIV education sessions for inmates at ten men's prisons. With funding from Burroughs-Wellcome, the program is led by two HIV-positive educators and covers prevention, testing, drug therapies for HIV disease, and support and treatment following release. Inmates at all ten prisons are able to ask questions using telephone hookups. A similar program has been presented for female inmates in Florida (Florida Department of Corrections, 1993).

Inmate Peer Programs. As suggested above, noninmates can certainly provide effective HIV education programs if they are carefully chosen for the ability to develop rapport with, and win the trust of, the audience. However, peer-based programs do offer a number of advantages. They can be implemented at little cost to the correctional system, since inmates provide most of the labor. Moreover, provided they are carefully selected and thoroughly trained, peer educators may be more credible with inmates and more likely to speak in terms relevant and understandable to inmates. Peer educators are also able to do substantial informal one-on-one outreach and support in the yard and other areas of the facility, in addition to conducting formal education, counseling, and support groups, and can be available on a twenty-four-hour basis.

Despite these advantages, inmate peer education programs on HIV are offered in only 35 percent of state/federal prison systems and only 7 percent of responding city/county jail systems. These percentages, based on central office responses, showed little change since the 1992–1993 NIJ/CDC survey.

A New York inmate who has worked to establish peer education programs in four different state prisons noted that it is really a "two-front" effort. The inmates themselves are often seriously divided along ethnic and racial lines; some are hostile to persons with HIV and to all efforts to address the problem of HIV, whether offered by persons with HIV or not. At the same time, the prison administration must be convinced of the value and importance of peer education programs. This is complicated by the often inherent suspicion of and opposition to inmate organization and inmate-initiated programs (Mahon, 1994b). This New York inmate reported meeting significant resistance from facility administrators. On several occasions, he was transferred to another facility just as he was beginning to get a peer program underway. (Correctional officials indicate that these transfers were routine, based on his high escape risk, and had nothing to do with his efforts to organize peer programs.) Currently, there are peer programs of varying levels of activity at about eight of sixty-eight New York State prisons (anonymous inmate, personal communication, November 10, 1994). These include the well-known and exemplary AIDS Counseling and Education (ACE) program at the Bedford Hills women's facility (described in detail below) and the PACE program at Eastern men's facility. The success and visibility of the ACE program spawned programs in other facilities and encouraged some correctional administrators to support peer programs.

Inmates and staff have both raised issues of confidentiality in opposition to peer programs. Concerns have been expressed that inmates' HIV status may be compromised through contact with peer educators or peer counselors. This could occur directly if the peer educators divulge information, or indirectly by other inmates' observing interactions between peer educators and HIV-infected inmates. The medical director at the Federal Penitentiary in Atlanta asserted that peer HIV counseling would result in putting a bulls-eye on inmates seen associating with the counselors. Staff at the Federal Bureau of Prisons' Metropolitan Correctional Center in Miami have not permitted peer programs for similar reasons (U.S. Penitentiary, Atlanta, personal communication, November 12, 1994; Metropolitan Correctional Center, Miami, personal communication, November 12, 1994).

Inmate peer educators in Oregon and elsewhere acknowledge that confidentiality is a serious issue. As a result, Oregon inmates cannot do pretest and posttest counseling but are firmly committed to maintaining confidentiality and to ending discrimination against persons with HIV (peer educators of Project O.A.S.I.S., Oregon State Penitentiary, personal communication, September 19, 1994). All peer programs must address this issue with sensitivity and care. The recently initiated inmate HIV peer education programs described below illustrate approaches that have worked well across a variety of correctional systems. As revealed in these examples, key ingredients of an effective HIV peer education program appear to be active support and collaboration of facility administrators, use of a variety of formats and vehicles for education and prevention messages, and availability of ad hoc, one-on-one contact as well as more formal and structured sessions.

ACE: An Exemplary Peer Education and Support Program for Women. Female inmates at New York's Bedford Hills Correctional Facility initiated the ACE (AIDS Counseling and Education) program in 1989 as a result of fears about HIV transmission and concerns about HIV-infected inmates' being stigmatized. Some women in the facility saw a need for AIDS counseling and education. Inmates manage the program, which offers inmate-to-inmate education, support groups, advocacy, and counseling. ACE counselors are certified by the state education department, and two civilians act as liaisons between the inmates and outside sources of funding and materials. However, the inmates themselves provide the HIV education and training inside the facility. This includes training of correctional staff, which has been well received. Indeed, after meeting with some initial resistance from the facility administration, ACE now enjoys the full support of the administration and the State Department of Correctional Services (Boudin & Clark, 1990).

The ACE program has its own office in the prison. The office is open Monday through Friday and every other Saturday, and it maintains an extensive resource library for inmates. There are twenty-five to thirty ACE members and two nonprisoners associated with the program (L. Mastroieni, ACE program, Bedford Hills Correctional Facility, personal communication, March 20, 1993).

As the ACE program has evolved, some of its original goals have been achieved. One of the initial goals was improvement of housing and environmental conditions for women with HIV disease. As a result of ACE's efforts, the infirmary is clean and much brightened by murals that inmates and ACE workers have painted.

ACE workers also organize recreational activities and AIDS education sessions within the infirmary.

The ACE program began in response to fear and misinformation about HIV transmission. Now every inmate has heard about AIDS from ACE members. The ACE program has educated hundreds of inmates. ACE members informally greet all new inmates. They introduce new inmates to ACE and invite them to an orientation. ACE's services are available to all inmates regardless of HIV status.

Various bilingual programs are offered by ACE, including medical advocacy, individual counseling, peer support and counseling, support groups for people with AIDS, seminars for those interested in becoming ACE members, and video discussion groups. ACE groups include spontaneous discussions and scheduled groups. Support groups meet daily with anywhere from two to twenty-five participants, reflecting the diversity of the inmate population. Topics discussed include living with AIDS, family issues, and relationships. Any topic that interests group participants is explored.

Medical advocacy is an important service, especially for Spanish-speaking clients. Bilingual ACE counselors accompany the inmates to medical appointments to ensure that they understand prescription information, HIV test results, and other medical issues. Like many of ACE's services, medical advocacy was initiated in response to inmates' stated needs.

There is also a community-based component of ACE (called ACE-OUT) that provides supportive services, including a "buddy" program and intensive case management for former inmates with HIV. ACE works with the Women's Prison Association to help place women in safe environments. ACE also helps women obtain social services, provides them with referrals, and updates their medical forms.

Oregon Sate Penitentiary: Project O.A.S.I.S (Oregon AIDS Support [Inmate] Services). Project O.A.S.I.S. was founded in 1994 by an inmate who became concerned after hearing many inaccurate statements about HIV from other inmates in the facility. With the support and close collaboration of a counselor from Correctional Treatment Services, O.A.S.I.S. initiated a number of programs and services including HIV workshops, one-on-one education and support, and referrals. Plans for the future include a buddy program for inmates with HIV/AIDS, a display of panels from the AIDS Quilt with associated educational programs, and development of HIV education videos. Currently, four highly dedicated and committed inmates are involved in the O.A.S.I.S. program; the group has applied for official recognition as a "special-interest inmate group" (O.A.S.I.S. members, personal communication, September 19, 1994).

A series of three one-hour sessions is offered each quarter as part of the regular school program in the prison. Topics include basic facts on HIV and its transmission and treatment, as well as practical guidance on condom use and cleaning of injection equipment. Four series were held during 1994, with an average attendance of twelve. A training manual and participant's workbook are being prepared.

One-on-one outreach, education, and support occurs in the yard and other parts of the prison. According to members of O.A.S.I.S., they provide support to a number of HIV-infected inmates who are too mistrustful to access the correctional system's health services. The peer team provides counseling, referrals to services both within and outside the facility (for those about to be released), and other services that help to free Correctional Treatment Services providers to do more pretest and posttest counseling.

Louisiana State Penitentiary, Angola: HIV/AIDS Peer Education Program. This program, founded in October 1993, has a staff of four inmate volunteers who received training from the state health department. All of these inmate peer educators have other prison jobs. Peer educators at Angola conduct weekly HIV education sessions for incoming inmates. One serious, but perhaps not uncommon, limitation is placed on this education by the prison administration: it is not allowed to cover specific safer-sex techniques (S. Hager, infection control coordinator, Louisiana State Penitentiary, personal communication, December 15, 1994).

In addition to the weekly sessions, the program has developed some innovative features, including almost weekly presentation of interviews and discussions of HIV issues on the facility's FM radio station (the only inmate-run station licensed by the Federal Communications Commission in the nation); working with the Angola

Drama Club (whose members have been trained as peer educators) to produce "The Enemy Within," a play on HIV written by one of the inmates; writing numerous articles for outside publications; speaking at other correctional facilities and other organizations in the community; and holding an all-day conference on HIV/AIDS at Angola in October 1994, attended by about three hundred persons from inside and outside the prison (S. Hager, personal communication, 1995). A second conference was held in November 1995.

The 1994 conference included welcoming remarks by the warden; sessions led by facility professional staff on HIV peer education programs, the epidemiology of HIV/AIDS at Angola, and medical treatment of inmates with HIV/AIDS; sessions led by peer educators ("The Impact of Life Sentences on HIV/AIDS in Prison," "The Pros and Cons of Segregating HIV-Infected Inmates," "HIV/AIDS: Double Impact Workable Solutions," "Living with HIV in Prison," and "Leaving the Penitentiary with HIV Infection"); and a presentation of the Drama Club's play on HIV in prisons. Peer educator Andrew Joseph told of how a life sentence and other pressures of prison life can engender carelessness about high-risk behavior. According to Joseph, some "lifers" "figure they will not get out of prison, so why should they care how they die? They begin to figure that it is better to die doing something that brings enjoyment to them than to waste away in prison and die of old age without family and friends." As a way of attempting to create a semblance of "normalcy in an abnormal place," Joseph and the peer education team strongly favor initiation of conjugal visits for inmates (Joseph, 1994; Schlichtman, 1994).

In "Double Impact Workable Solutions," peer educator G. Ashanti Witherspoon cogently described the impact of HIV/AIDS within the prison and outside, as inmates return to the community, and the generally inadequate correctional response in terms of medical care, education, and peer counseling. Witherspoon proposed a solution consisting of comprehensive peer education for inmates, education for correctional staff and administrators, and cooperation among correctional staff, health departments, and community-based organizations to develop effective HIV services for inmates that are also sensitive to the security concerns of correctional officials. Witherspoon described some of the programs at Angola, including incorporation of HIV issues into the inmate-run CPR training program (Witherspoon, 1994).

Theortic "Bojack" Givens outlined a discharge planning program under development by the peer educators at Angola that they hope will be implemented at all Louisiana prisons. This is part of the peer education team's overall effort to close the gaps among "those who make things happen; those who watch things happen; and those who ask what happened" (Givens, 1994). With the inspiration and encouragement of the Angola program, inmates at Avoyelles Correctional Center, another men's prison in Louisiana, recently began an HIV peer education program.

California Medical Facility, Vacaville: HIV Peer Education Program. California Medical Facility, Vacaville, is one of the largest correctional facilities in the United States. It houses most of the system's known male HIV-infected inmates. Several different peer education programs have existed at Vacaville over the years. A recent program, described here, seemed the most solid until it was abruptly terminated by the Department of Corrections.

The HIV peer education program was an official program of the Vacaville facility, with detailed policies and procedures, and a psychiatric social worker—a paid staff member of the prison—supervising the six inmate peer educators. These positions were paid inmate jobs. Peer educators were to receive at least four hours of training each month. The educators reflected the diversity of the inmate population: three black, three Hispanic, and three white. The threefold mission of the peer program was to work toward elimination of HIV transmission and reinfection within the facility, increase understanding of HIV/AIDS and compassion for inmates living with HIV, and create a "norm devaluing high-risk behaviors" (HIV Peer Education Program, 1993).

To achieve these goals, the program adopted a multimedia strategy, involving live presentations, guest speakers, videos, slides, audiocassettes, role plays, storytelling, drama, posters, and a resource library. Because of the program's conviction that "learning takes place over time," sessions were presented on an ongoing basis every month.

Topics covered in monthly sessions included psychosocial issues in living with HIV, self-esteem and taking responsibility for one's behaviors, proper condom use, proper procedures for cleaning needles and injection material, relapse prevention, and maintaining behavior change. Although sessions included information on safer sex and safer injection practices, each was preceded by a statement that drug use, tattooing, condoms, and sexual activity are prohibited in prison and that the education is not intended to encourage any prohibited practices.

In addition to the monthly education sessions, the peer program at Vacaville offered on-call initial education for all new arrivals at the facility and counseling for HIV-infected inmates and those concerned about high-risk behavior or HIV antibody testing. The program emphasized the facts about HIV and the importance of treating HIV-infected persons with respect and compassion. The texts of two posters developed by the program reflected these themes:

> Public Notice: As of 1993, there have been 194,334 AIDS-related deaths in the United States. As of 1993, there has been no documented case of a person contracting the disease by eating food prepared or served by a[n] HIV positive person. [Ironically, . . .
> a recent court decision allowed the California Department of Corrections to exclude HIV-infected inmates from food service jobs on the ground that their presence in such jobs might cause a riot. This suggests the persistence of some aspects of HIV-related misinformation in correctional facilities.]

> Don't condemn those with HIV or AIDS. Condemn those who would turn their backs on those with HIV or AIDS.

Audiovisual and Written Materials

Eighty-eight percent of state/federal systems and 66 percent of city/county systems reported employing videos and other audiovisual materials in HIV education programs. Ninety-four percent of prison systems and 72 percent of responding jail systems said they distributed written materials on HIV.

Materials used in HIV education and prevention programs must be understandable and accessible to the target populations and sensitive to diverse cultures and gender groups. The reported mean reading level for HIV materials used in prison and jail systems was seventh grade, which seems appropriate. Seventy-one percent of state/federal systems reported using written materials on HIV specifically addressed to women, while 61 percent of prison systems said they had materials specifically prepared for Hispanics, 31 percent for blacks, and 18 percent for Asian Americans. The figures for city/county jail systems were: women 66 percent, Hispanics 66 percent, blacks 55 percent, and Asian Americans 24 percent.

HIV Precautionary and Preventive Measures

Responding effectively to HIV/AIDS within correctional facilities requires instituting reasonable procedures to protect inmates and staff from HIV infection. However, implementing constructive policies often involves balancing conflicting demands. A key principle in this effort is that whatever precautionary and preventive measures are instituted be consistent with educational messages provided to inmates and staff about HIV/AIDS. Policies or procedures that conflict with or go beyond educational messages may cause unnecessary fear and increased mistrust of correctional authorities.

Infection Control Based on Universal Precautions

Very few correctional systems report policies of notifying correctional officers of inmates' HIV status. These policies are still under debate. Some correctional officers and unions believe that they need, and should have access to, this information in order to protect themselves on the job. Opponents of disclosure policies generally point to two problems. The first is that no practicable testing program could ever ensure that all HIV-infected inmates are known. Because the widely available tests detect only the presence of antibodies to HIV, and not the virus itself, there can be a window period of up to six months and sometimes longer during which someone who is HIV-infected may still test negative. However, programs of mandatory testing and notification might create the illusion that all infected people had been identified; this in turn could foster a false sense of security. Second, particularly in systems with many HIV-infected persons, it would be easy to forget or confuse who is HIV positive.

The best alternative to a disclosure policy is the principle of "universal precautions." Universal precautions treat all people as if they are infected. This means avoiding unprotected contact with body fluids that are considered potentially infective, especially blood and semen. Revised guidelines from CDC state that universal precautions are not necessary for contact with saliva, tears, sweat, vomitus, urine, or feces, unless they contain visible blood (Centers for Disease Control, 1988b).

Universal precautions, long recommended by the CDC for health care settings, apply equally well to correctional and law enforcement settings. The precautions should be practiced by both staff and inmates in correctional facilities as a sound approach to prevention of all blood-borne infectious diseases, including hepatitis B and C. CDC issued extensive guidelines regarding HIV transmission and prevention for health care and emergency workers in 1989. These include recommendations for use of protective equipment, such as gloves and CPR masks, and for disposal of needles and other "sharps," body and cell searches, handling of infectious materials, and cleaning up of spills. Procedures to follow once an exposure has occurred are also specified; these include medical protocols and procedures for documenting incidents (Centers for Disease Control, 1989).

There is evidence, however, that despite strong recommendations and their embodiment in written policy, universal precautions are not well implemented in at least some corrections settings. Surveillance of possible occupational exposures to HIV in a state correctional system identified 166 incidents, including needle sticks, nonintact skin exposures, and mucous membrane exposures. Although no HIV infections occurred as a result of these incidents, CDC concluded that over half of the exposures could have been prevented had personal protective equipment been used (Centers for Disease Control, 1992c).

Regulations issued by the Occupational Safety and Health Administration (OSHA) in December 1991 gave full legal force to universal precautions in health care, correctional, and other work settings. Under these regulations, employers are required to:

- Establish written exposure control plans
- Identify and train workers who face potential exposure to blood-borne pathogens and tuberculosis
- Provide necessary infection control equipment
- Offer free hepatitis B vaccinations and PPD skin testing for tuberculosis infection
- Provide evaluation and follow-up services to any employees who have had potential exposures

[Occupational Safety and Health Administration, 1994]

Detailed infection control policies and procedures, many of which are based on CDC's guidelines and universal precautions, have been adopted by many correctional systems. The policies and procedures in these systems must also be consistent with OSHA regulations.

Although CDC guidelines and OSHA regulations call for the implementation of universal precautions, no set of written policies or procedures can cover all contingencies, particularly in unpredictable environments such as prisons and jails. Situations faced by law enforcement and correctional personnel often require an immediate response. In exigent situations, officers and other staff must use their judgment in the application of universal precautions. However, infection control policies can provide general guidance and inform decisions made by correctional staff. Training is also essential, so staff have a clear understanding of high-risk incidents and the opportunity to discuss possible situations and appropriate responses.

Availability of Barrier Protection

Many correctional systems include discussions of safer sex practices in their HIV educational programs. In the vast majority of correctional systems, however, the means to put these messages into practice are not officially provided.

The number of systems that make condoms available to inmates has remained stable for several years. Mississippi's state system reported that they do distribute condoms, and at one male facility in Parchman condoms are sold in the canteen. However, at the Central Mississippi Correctional Facility, condoms are currently not distributed to inmates. Staff at this facility have discussed the possibility of distributing condoms through the pharmacy or through an education program. Vermont's is the only other state system that distributes condoms.

No systems have begun distributing condoms since the 1992 NIJ/CDC survey. The San Francisco, Philadelphia, New York City, and Washington, D.C., jail systems also distribute condoms. Further, one other jail system reported making condoms available to inmates in practice, although there is no official policy authorizing distribution of condoms. The medical director of this jail system reported that he was motivated by clear public health needs, although disclosure of the practice would likely provoke public disapproval. Condom availability has also been instituted in all Canadian federal prisons and some provincial prisons (Expert Committee on AIDS and Prisons, 1994). Six state correctional systems in the United States, including the New York State system, make condoms available for conjugal visits.

The details of condom distribution vary by correctional system. Inmates at the Mississippi State Penitentiary in Parchman can buy unlimited supplies of condoms at the canteen for 25 cents each. However, most systems tie condom distribution to health services or HIV education. In New York City, inmates are limited to one condom per medical visit and are supposed to be counseled by medical staff before receiving a condom. In Vermont, condoms are available through health services with counseling in most instances, but they are sometimes also made available in health services offices without counseling. In at least one Vermont institution, lubricant is provided with condoms.

Condoms are available at HIV/AIDS educational programs in San Francisco, and at HIV antibody test counseling sessions or during sick call in Philadelphia. Condoms are available in the infirmary and at counseling and education sessions in District of Columbia jails (M. Campbell, District of Columbia Department of Corrections, personal communication, April 1993). The number of condoms distributed to inmates annually varies widely by correctional system and is no doubt related to the method of distribution. In New York City, where condoms are only available after counseling, about twelve hundred condoms are distributed annually. By contrast, in San Francisco, condoms are available to all who participate in HIV education programs, and about ten thousand condoms are distributed each year (Greenberg & Halperin, 1994).

In the San Francisco and District of Columbia jail systems, HIV prevention for women is specifically addressed by making dental dams available. These are squares of latex that can be used as barrier protection for oral-genital sex between women.

The Debate over Condom Availability

Correctional medical staff often advocate condom availability while correctional administrators and security staff oppose it. This disagreement reflects differing perspectives. Health care workers view corrections from the public health model, which acknowledges that sex takes place in prison and stresses the need to prevent HIV transmission. On the other hand, correctional officials tend to emphasize security and adherence to regulations. They worry that condom distribution would signal an acceptance of sex within the institution, which is proscribed, and that condoms might be used as weapons or to conceal drugs or other contraband. Some correctional medical staff have implemented what they consider appropriate public health measures, such as distribution of condoms, even when this was prohibited by the correctional system ("Prisons' Care Systems Swamped," 1990).

In Vermont, the condom availability policy was actually championed at first by a deputy superintendent of one of the facilities. He believed at the time, and continues to believe, that "good public health policy is good correctional policy." According to this correctional administrator, sex happens in prisons and it would be irresponsible not to make protection available (staff of Chittenden Regional Correctional Center, South Burlington, Vermont); Northwest State Correctional Facility, Swanton, Vermont; personal communications, November 8, 1994).

In the systems with condom availability, there have been few if any problems with condoms being used as weapons or for smuggling contraband, despite suggestions by opponents that this would occur. A hospital administrator at the Mississippi State prison in Parchman recalled only one incident when a condom was used for smuggling contraband (Walker, 1992). In Vermont, after an initial period of some heightened interest and controversy, condom distribution became routine and was no longer an issue. Vermont officials report few if any problems with misuse of condoms for smuggling contraband or for weapons, and they suggest that there is no evidence of an increase in sexual activity or undesirable behavior since the condom policy was instituted. In a survey of over four hundred officers in Canada's federal prison system, 82 percent reported that condom availability had created no problems in their facilities (Expert Committee on AIDS and Prisons, 1994).

Bleach and Needle Availability

Many correctional systems include information on safer injection practices in their education and counseling. However, only two systems have policies for provision of bleach, and no systems distribute needles. Since injection drug use is illegal in prison and in the outside community, correctional officials conclude that distributing bleach or needles would condone illegal activity. Moreover, needles and bleach do pose serious security and safety risks in correctional facilities. Still, needles are present in many facilities, and their scarcity tends to foster sharing and other risky practices. A British study found that although needle use was rarer in prisons than on the street, it tended to be riskier when it did occur (Turnbull & Dolan, 1992). A Scottish study provides further indication of high risk with injection drug use in prisons. Of forty-three inmates in Glenochil prison who admitted to injection drug use at some time in their lives but not while in prison, thirty-four were tested for HIV antibody and none were positive. By contrast, twelve of twenty-five (44 percent) of inmates who admitted to injecting drugs in prison tested HIV seropositive (Taylor et al., 1995).

In the United States, among the correctional systems responding to the 1994 NIJ/CDC survey, only the San Francisco jail systems officially makes bleach available for cleaning drug injection material. A pilot program of bleach distribution is being implemented in Canada, and the Canadian Expert Committee on AIDS and Prisons recommends making small quantities of full-strength bleach "easily and discreetly accessible" to inmates (Expert Committee on AIDS and Prisons, 1994). However, bleach is available for general cleaning purposes in many systems, and some inmates may have de facto access to bleach for needle cleaning even in the absence of policies explicitly permitting this.

Recent research has shown that bleach may not be fully effective for disinfecting injection equipment unless its use carefully follows correct procedure. The CDC's revised procedure calls for rinsing with clean water, then with full-strength bleach, then with clean water again at least three times, shaking the syringe for thirty seconds during each rinsing. Although proper cleaning with bleach does significantly reduce the risk of HIV transmission, the only way to be certain that there is no infected blood in a needle or syringe is to use new sterile equipment every time. Bleach is only recommended "when no other safer options are available" (Centers for Disease Control and Prevention, 1993).

Although there are no needle exchange programs in prisons in the United States, a Swiss prison has started a pilot needle exchange program. The medical officer of another prison in that country instituted needle exchange on his own, without the approval of the correctional authorities. Inmates at the first Swiss prison, Hindelbank Institution for Women, can exchange used needles and syringes for sterile ones at automatic dispensers throughout the institution. They can also receive counseling and education on HIV (Nelles & Harding, 1995; Jurgens, 1994b). Some argue that providing needles to inmates condones illegal activity and creates safety risks within an institution. However, Martin Lachat, interim director of the Hindelbank Institution for Women, commented: "The transmission of HIV or any other serious disease cannot be tolerated. Given that all we can do is restrict, not suppress, the entry of drugs, we feel it is our responsibility to at least provide sterile syringes to inmates. The ambiguity of our mandate leads to a contradiction that we have to live with" (Nelles & Harding, 1995; Jurgens, 1994b).

The Canadian Expert Committee on AIDS and Prisons recommended further research, including scientifically valid pilot studies, on needle exchange in prisons (Expert Committee on AIDS and Prisons, 1994).

HIV and STD Testing, Counseling, Confidentiality, and Disclosure Policies

A fairly stable list of correctional systems continues to have policies for mandatory HIV antibody testing of inmates. In some instances, however, the justification for this policy has shifted from one based on prevention of transmission (even, oddly, in the absence of an associated segregation policy) to one more grounded in medical intervention. Although mandatory testing could, in theory, increase access to diagnosis and treatment, most systems have found it preferable to pursue the goals of medical intervention and treatment in the context of voluntary or on-request testing policies. The CDC continues to help fund confidential HIV counseling and testing services in numerous correctional facilities through its cooperative agreements with public health departments.

HIV Antibody Testing Policies

Table 5.3 shows that mandatory HIV testing continues to be the policy of a minority of state/federal prison systems, but it is an apparently stable minority. For the first time, the 1994 survey

Table 5.3. HIV Antibody Testing of Inmates, Hierarchical Categorization, 1994[a].

Procedure	U.S. State/Federal Prison Systems (n = 51)		U.S. City/County Jail Systems (n = 29)	
	n	%	n	%
Mandatory mass screening (all incoming inmates, current inmates, and/ or inmates at release)	17	33	0	0
Voluntary/inmate request testing	30	59	28	97
Testing if clinical indications[b]	4	8	1	3
Total	51	100	29	100

[a] Includes actual and planned policies. This is a hierarchical categorization: jurisdictions that do mass screening are placed in the uppermost category, regardless of whether they also test for other purposes; jurisdictions that offer voluntary or on-request screening are placed in the voluntary category regardless of whether they also test when clinically indicated.

[b] In this table, clinical indications include lowered CD4 (T4) counts, opportunistic infections, TB positivity, or active TB.

Source: NIJ/CDC questionnaire responses.

included pregnant females as a separate category for mandatory HIV testing. Thirteen state systems (26 percent) reported mandatory testing for pregnant women. None of the responding city/county systems reported mandatory testing of pregnant inmates.

Mandatory Screening. Table 5.4 lists the sixteen state prison systems that, along with the Federal Bureau of Prisons, report mandatory mass HIV screening of inmates at intake or release. Six of these state systems test at both times, while the Federal Bureau of Prisons reports mandatory testing only at release. Due to the rapid turnover of inmates in jails, it is not surprising that none of the responding city/county jail systems reports mandatory mass screening policies. High turnover rates make the logistics of mass screening very difficult. There has been no change in the number of systems reporting mandatory screening since the 1992 NIJ/CDC survey.

Although sixteen prison systems report HIV screening at intake, the Alabama and Mississippi state systems remain the only two systems to segregate all known HIV-infected inmates. Housing policies are discussed later in this chapter.

Voluntary/On-Request Testing. A large percentage of prison and jail systems offer HIV testing to inmates on request. In fact, among city/county systems, voluntary or on-request testing is the most frequently reported basis of testing. Dr. Jan Diamond, a physician who formerly worked in the California prison system, argues strongly for encouragement of voluntary inmate HIV testing because it is "an important way to reach a disenfranchised population . . . who otherwise receive little HIV intervention or health care" (Diamond, 1994).

Successful encouragement of voluntary inmate testing may be challenging. Studies in New York State prisons show higher rates of HIV seropositivity in blinded epidemiologic studies representative of the entire inmate population than among those who came forward for voluntary testing. The apparent reluctance of HIV-positive individuals to be tested is at variance with the assumption that individuals who are at high risk for HIV infection will come forward for testing, particularly if they believe that they can benefit from early medical intervention. For both medical and psycho-

Table 5.4. Correctional Systems Conducting Mandatory Screening of Inmates, June–December 1994a.

U.S. State/Federal Prison Systems (n = 51)	U.S. City/County Jail Systems (n = 29)
Federal Bureau of Prisons	none
Alabama	
Colorado	
Georgia	
Idaho	
Iowa	
Michigan	
Mississippi	
Missouri	
Nebraska	
Nevada	
New Hampshire	
North Dakota	
Oklahoma	
Rhode Island	
Utah	
Wyoming	

a Defined as mandatory HIV antibody testing, generally identity-linked, of all new inmates, all releasees, and/or all current inmates, regardless of whether they show clinical indications of HIV infection. In terms of correctional policy, this type of testing differs in purpose and method from blinded epidemiological studies. Blinded studies are anonymous (not identity-linked) screenings intended to assess seroprevalence rates in a particular population.

Source: NIJ/CDC questionnaire responses.

logical reasons, this assumption may be flawed. First, recent research suggests that early intervention with ZDV is probably ineffective in lengthening survival with AIDS. Second, whether or not they have considered the benefits of early medical intervention, many individuals may feel that it is psychologically easier not to know their HIV status: put simply, they do not want any bad news. In a Maryland study of voluntary testing, in which about half of the inmates chose to be tested, the most common reason for declining testing was fear of a positive result (Behrendt et al., 1994). A nurse at a Vermont prison echoed this conclusion (L. McMorrow, Northwest State Correctional Facility, personal communication, November 8, 1994).

Despite the discouraging news about early treatment with ZDV, there may be other early interventions useful for at least some who learn their HIV status. These include prophylaxis for *Pneumocystis carinii pneumonia* (PCP) or other opportunistic infections associated with HIV infection, immunizations, and counseling regarding diet and food preparation to avoid food-borne pathogens.

A combination of mass HIV education, followed up with intensive counseling focusing on individuals who self-identify as high-risk, may be a more effective means of getting inmates to volunteer for HIV testing (LaChance-McCullough et al., 1994). Research done in the New York City jail system provides support for this strategy (Florio, Bellini, Safyer, & Fletcher, 1992).

Diamond recommended the following methods of maximizing acceptance of voluntary testing:

• Using noncorrectional staff for counseling and testing
• Maintaining confidentiality if at all possible
• Considering the use of anonymous testing
• Providing follow-up after testing, with high-quality counseling, education, and medical care
 [Diamond, 1994]

Confidentiality and Disclosure of HIV Status

One of the best ways to maximize acceptance of testing by those most at risk for HIV is to ensure that confidentiality of results is protected. In correctional settings, this poses great challenges. The majority of prison and jail systems have policies against notifying correctional staff, other than medical staff, of inmates' HIV status. Policies permitting disclosure to nonmedical staff usually limit this to central office or institutional management staff. Indeed, policies for disclosure to such staff declined among state and federal systems by 12 percent and 14 percent respectively since the 1992 NIJ/CDC survey. In 1994, only four state systems (8 percent) and four responding city/county systems (15 percent) reported policies for notifying line correctional officers of inmates' HIV status. The validation study revealed a high rate of facilities' compliance with central office policies against notification of correctional officers.

According to the 1994 NIJ/CDC survey, the most commonly notified parties, as a matter of official policy, are the inmate, the medical staff, and the public health department. Next most common is notification of sexual partners. A partner notification policy might mean that the inmate notifies the partner(s) directly, that correctional officials notify the partner(s), or that public health authorities are notified and they follow up with the partner(s). About 90 percent of the state/federal systems and 75 percent of city/county systems use two or more methods of notification. In such cases, notification of sexual partner(s) is not left entirely up to the inmate.

Beyond officially stated policies at the system or facility level, actually maintaining confidentiality of HIV-related and other sensitive information is extremely difficult in a correctional setting. One state system uniformly "flags" with a prominent sticker the medical records of inmates who are infected with blood-borne diseases. Although official policy does not require or authorize notification, medical staff practice may provide inmates or correctional staff with opportunities to learn confidential information.

Flagging or obvious coding of medical records has become relatively uncommon, but other means of unofficial disclosure of HIV status remain in the normal course of correctional life. Even without obvious flagging of records, medical staff or inmates working in medical units have access to the information and may disclose it. In part because of high levels of enforced idleness among inmates, prison gossip networks and rumor mills are extremely active. Despite official policies, many correctional officers and inmates believe they are entitled to know who is HIV-infected. Correctional officers have substantial power and can use it to obtain information. In short, official policies will only protect confidentiality if they are enforced through vigilant monitoring.

HIV Pretest/Posttest Counseling

Pretest and posttest counseling are critical components of HIV programs in correctional facilities. Over half of all correctional systems reported providing HIV counseling in all of their facilities. Sixteen percent of state/federal systems and 13 percent of city/county systems report that less than 50 percent of their facilities are providing counseling. On average, 78 percent of facilities in state/federal and city/county systems are reportedly providing counseling.

Pretest and posttest counseling should be provided on an individual basis. However, many correctional systems simply do not have sufficient staff to offer individual pretest counseling, and therefore they conduct this counseling in groups. It is absolutely essential that posttest counseling be given individually; almost all correctional systems report this to be their policy. However, as with confidentiality, policy does not always translate into practice. There continue to be numerous allegations regarding failure to conduct counseling with inmates when tests are negative (thereby losing an important education opportunity) and insensitive and inappropriate methods of notifying seropositive inmates.

Housing Policies

Since the first NIJ survey was conducted in 1985, there has been a marked trend away from policies calling for the segregation of inmates with HIV infection and AIDS. Table 5.5 shows the steady decline in the number of state/federal prison systems reporting segregation of inmates with AIDS and asymptomatic HIV infection. In 1985, thirty-eight (75 percent) of the prison systems reported segregating inmates with AIDS and eight systems (16 percent) reported segregating inmates with asymptomatic HIV (then called HTLV-III) infection. By 1994, the numbers had shrunk to four and two systems respectively.

This trend resulted from a steady erosion of the view that segregation represents an effective and prudent method of preventing transmission of HIV. At the same time, alleviation of the earlier levels of hostility and even hysteria surrounding inmates with HIV disease have rendered it much more feasible for them to be housed in the general population of correctional facilities.

Table 5.5. Decline of Segregation Policies in State/Federal Systems ($n = 51$), 1985–1994.

| | Systems with Segregation Policies | | | |
| | HIV-Infected Inmates | | Inmates with AIDS | |
Years	n	%	n	%
1985	8	16	38	75
1986	8	16	30	59
1987	5	10	41	80
1988	6	12	20	39
1989	4	8	16	31
1990	4	8	9	18
1992	2	4	5	10
1994	2	4	4	8

Source: NIJ/CDC questionnaire responses.

The same two state prison systems, those in Alabama and Mississippi, that reported segregating all known HIV-infected inmates in 1992 still reported such a policy in 1994. Alabama's segregation policy is the subject of a continuing lawsuit.

No city/county jail systems responding to the 1994 NIJ/CDC survey reported segregating inmates with HIV disease. While segregation policies have continued to lose favor, there was some shift between the 1992 and 1994 surveys from policies calling for general population housing to those calling for case-by-case decisions. Some of this apparent shift may be due to respondents' uncertainty about the meaning of the categories, that is, a policy for presumptive general population housing of inmates with HIV may be hard to distinguish from a policy in which decisions are made on a case-by-case basis. At the same time, there may also have been some real spread of the view that a case-by-case decision-making policy offers the best way to address the medical and psychosocial needs of inmates with HIV disease.

The real complexity of policies regarding housing and programming for inmates with HIV, particularly in large systems with

HIV-infected inmates in multiple facilities, is well illustrated by the situation in the California state correctional system. The following discussion is based on a December 1994 interview with Matthew Coles, formerly with the American Civil Liberties Union Foundation of Northern California (personal communication, December, 1994).

A 1990 consent decree in the case of *Gates* v. *Deukmejian,* which had challenged the state's policy of segregating all known male HIV-infected inmates in a closed wing at California Medical Facility, Vacaville, established a pilot program of partial integration for selected inmates (*Gates* v. *Deukmejian,* 1990). These inmates continued to live in a separate wing but could participate in educational and work programs with the general population of the facility. The pilot program was to be monitored and either expanded or adjusted, based on performance.

Over time, a dual system has been established at Vacaville and San Quentin, with open units (separate housing and integrated programming as in the original pilot program) and closed units (continued separate housing and programming). Inmates with documented histories of high-risk behavior (participation in anal intercourse, oral sex, or assault involving potential blood exposure to another) within the past year and those for whom there is "reasonable cause to believe" they will engage in such behaviors are excluded from assignment to an open unit (*Gates* v. *Rowland,* 1994). At Vacaville and San Quentin there is no full integration of known HIV-infected inmates into the general population, although there are believed to be numerous inmates whose infection is not known to the correctional department and who remain in general-population housing and programming. The plaintiff's attorneys in the Gates case have not fought to end segregated housing for HIV-infected inmates at Vacaville, because the vast majority of these inmates want this to continue. Matthew Coles, the former lead attorney, asserted that this is because the inmates with HIV feel safer being housed in the separate wing and believe they benefit from a stronger internal support system there. They are satisfied with this arrangement as long as they can participate in programs in the general population.

At the men's prison at San Luis Obispo, by contrast, known HIV-infected inmates live in the general population, but most are

double-celled together. The prison authorities will not knowingly
assign HIV-infected and non–HIV-infected inmates to be cell
mates.

Finally, at the women's prison at Frontera all three conditions
exist: closed unit, open unit, and general population housing. The
California situation shows how differing policies are known and
permitted to exist in different facilities.

Work Assignments and Other Programming

In most instances, inmates with HIV who live in the general population or have access to general-population programming are eligible for all work assignments and other programs. However, some
types of program assignments have continued to be controversial.
In California, participation by HIV-infected inmates in four types
of programming—work furloughs, medical services jobs, family visits, and food-service jobs—remained at issue at the time of the
agreement on housing units. Subsequently, correctional officials
allowed HIV-infected inmates to participate in work furloughs and
work in medical services jobs, but they have remained firm in their
opposition to family visits and food-service work assignments.

Indeed, assignment of inmates with HIV to food-service work
assignments has continued to provoke controversy in a number of
systems. In Arizona, a federal district court ruled out exclusion of
HIV-infected inmates from food-service assignments as a violation
of the Federal Rehabilitation Act, but this decision was subsequently overturned by the Ninth Circuit Court of Appeals on technical grounds (*Casey* v. *Lewis*, 1991, 1993). In California, the
correctional system's exclusion of HIV-infected inmates from food-
service jobs was also upheld by the Ninth Circuit Court of Appeals.
There was agreement regarding the lack of evidence of HIV transmission through food, but the court still accepted the correctional
department's position that assigning HIV-infected inmates to food-
service jobs might lead to prison riots and abuse of those inmates.
The Ninth Circuit Court's ruling overturned an earlier district
court opinion on the issue of food-service work assignments (*Gates*
v. *Rowland*, 1994).

Policies that exclude HIV-infected inmates from food-service
jobs or force them to eat on disposable dishes contradict and

undermine educational messages. If educational programs stress that HIV is not contracted through casual contact, including food and utensils, then inmates will question the necessity of excluding HIV-infected persons from food-service jobs. Likewise, they may wonder why disposable plates and utensils are used. Such concerns may lead to mistrust of the correct educational messages and breed fear about casual transmission of HIV. These policies may also break the confidentiality of HIV-infected inmates. Inmates can quickly deduce that anyone refused a food-service job or forced to use disposable utensils is HIV-infected ("Confidentiality Said Breached," 1990).

Conjugal Visits

Conjugal visits are available to inmates in only eight state/federal prison systems (16 percent). No city/county jail systems reported making conjugal visits available to inmates. In those systems with conjugal visit programs, five (10 percent of all state/federal systems) make these visits available to HIV-infected inmates. In 1991, the New York State correctional system reversed an earlier policy and opened conjugal visits to HIV-infected prisoners. As noted above, HIV-infected inmates in California continue to be excluded from conjugal visits. In Louisiana, inmate HIV peer educators have argued that instituting conjugal visits would reduce the sexual tension that leads to homosexual contact in prisons and often to high-risk sexual activity among inmates (Joseph, 1994).

Early and Compassionate Release

Since inmates in the advanced stages of AIDS and other terminal illnesses pose little threat to the community, it has commonly been argued that they should be afforded early release so that they can return to their families and communities and not be forced to die in prison. The 1994 NIJ/CDC survey reveals that thirty-one state/federal prison systems (61 percent) and eleven responding city/county jail systems (38 percent) have policies for early or compassionate release, and nineteen state/federal systems (37 percent) and seven city/county systems (24 percent) have policies for medical furlough of such inmates. A total of 214 inmates in twenty-two state/federal systems and 131 inmates in nine city/county systems have reportedly been released under such policies.

The hard-line political climate regarding treatment of criminals and the publicity surrounding crimes committed by inmates who were released through various programs have contributed to the difficulty of establishing and taking full advantage of early-release programs for terminally ill inmates. In Massachusetts, a medical parole bill was vetoed by the governor even though it included strong requirements for certification that the inmate to be released should pose no threat to the community.

At the same time, revisions to the New York State medical parole bill adopted in the spring of 1994 render that provision more likely to be used. The original legislation required a physician to make a judgment that the inmate was unlikely to commit further crimes if released. Very few physicians were willing to make such a nonmedical judgment. Under the legislative revisions, the physician is asked only to make a medical judgment that the prisoner's illness is terminal and results in severe restrictions of his or her ability to self-ambulate ("New Hope," 1994). Over fifty New York State inmates with AIDS or other terminal illnesses were released on medical parole during 1994, as opposed to a total of only six through January 1993. There is no evidence that any of these individuals committed serious crimes following their release.

In Maryland, as part of a comprehensive discharge planning program (discussed below), inmates with HIV/AIDS are identified for expedited medical parole and their cases are coordinated by a special staff of case managers and a nurse consultant. Under this program, the number of inmates receiving medical parole increased from eight in 1991 to twenty-three in 1993. None of the inmates released on medical parole has been reincarcerated for violent crimes (Boyle & Kummer, 1994).

Medical Care and Psychosocial Services

The provision of medical care and psychosocial services for inmates with HIV disease continue to pose challenges for correctional systems as the number of inmates requiring services increases and pressure on budgets is heightened. In the face of escalating costs and caseloads in HIV/AIDS and other health problems, many correctional systems are turning to contracted services and managed care approaches (McDonald, 1994). Inmates with HIV disease remain seriously underserved and are often treated with cruelty and insensitivity (A. Braudy, staff attorney, Massachusetts Correctional Legal Services, personal communication, November 17, 1994). Prisoners with AIDS are still sometimes relegated to the "care" of untrained, incompetent, and unconcerned staff, where they are permitted to die alone, without proper medical treatment or supportive services (Greenspan, 1994). It is also sad but true that many inmates are getting more and better medical and psychosocial services in prison than they ever got on the outside. Although the state of care for inmates with HIV disease still needs improving, most correctional systems have come a long way in making medical and psychosocial services available (T. Gagnon, Massachusetts Department of Public Health, personal communication, December 2, 1994). There is clearly a mixed pattern, with some systems providing better levels of care than others.

Particularly challenging areas in the realm of medical and psychosocial services, beyond escalating caseloads and budgetary pressures, include ongoing availability of therapeutic drugs, regular high-quality primary and specialty care (and the proper mix of these services), care for AIDS dementia and other neuropsychological manifestations of HIV disease, case management, follow-up and continuity of care, hospice care, access to clinical trials and experimental therapies, and appropriate nutritional supplements. Important aspects of adjunctive and psychosocial services include ongoing counseling and support, as well as substance abuse treatment. The Correctional Association of New York has offered a series of policy proposals for improving medical care for inmates with HIV/AIDS. These include the following:

- Standardized medical care policies and protocols
- Independent quality assurance
- Delivery of care by departments of health or private providers
- A primary health care model
- Expanded resources and support for correctional health care
- Minority, multilingual, and multicultural health staff
- High quality women's health care

- Access to AIDS-related clinical trials
- Training in neuropsychological symptoms

[AIDS in Prison Project, 1994]

Availability of Prophylactic and Therapeutic Drugs for Inmates with HIV Disease

The availability of zidovudine (ZDV) to inmates continues to be widespread in correctional systems throughout the United States. The 1994 NIJ/CDC survey reveals that ZDV is available in all responding correctional systems.

Although still less common in correctional care than ZDV, other antiretroviral drugs have become increasingly available to inmates with HIV/AIDS. Didanosine (ddI) is offered by 86 percent of state/federal systems and 96 percent of responding city/county systems. Didanosine is most commonly used when the patient is resistant or intolerant to ZDV, or when ZDV produces no clinical improvement.

Zalcitabine (ddC) is also most commonly used in cases of resistance or intolerance to ZDV, or when the CD4 count is 500 or lower with symptoms, or simply at the recommendation of the physician. Although the 1994 survey reveals that ddC is fairly widely available, 24 percent of state/federal systems and 18 percent of responding city/county systems do not offer this therapy to inmates with HIV disease.

Bactrim/Septra, now a much more commonly used prophylactic than aerosolized pentamidine for *Pneumocystis carinii pneumonia*, appears to be used most often when the patient's CD4 count is 200 or less (in 42 percent of state/federal and 37 percent city/county systems). This prophylactic therapy is available in 96 percent of state/federal systems and in all but one responding city/county system.

Access to Experimental Therapies and Clinical Trials

Access to both clinical trials and experimental therapies is still limited in prisons and jails. Just over one-quarter of state/federal systems (28 percent) offer experimental drugs to inmates with HIV disease (a 10 percent increase over 1992–1993), while only three of the responding city/county systems offer such access. The low rate of access in jail systems probably relates to the high turnover in these facilities.

After a long period of pessimism and seeming stagnation, there have recently been a number of promising developments in HIV treatment, including favorable results from various combination therapies and a new class of drugs called protease inhibitors. At this writing, it is not known how widely these new approaches are available to prisoners. Given experience, however, the likelihood is that these innovative treatments are largely unavailable to inmates.

Only six state/federal systems (12 percent)—Maryland, New York, Texas, Ohio, Virginia, and the Federal Bureau of Prisons—reported to the 1994 NIJ/CDC survey that they had inmates in clinical trials, most commonly Phase II and Phase III efficacy trials. This represented no change from the previous survey, conducted in 1992. While a number of other systems permit inmate participation in trials, such participation often poses logistical difficulties and involves additional cost. Inmate subjects must sometimes adhere to complicated regimens and must be transported to outside medical centers for follow-up appointments.

Psychosocial and Supportive Services

Some organizations working with prisoners with HIV cite an ongoing lack of "regular, sympathetic and compassionate treatment" in correctional facilities (A. Montgomery, Span, Inc., Prison to the Community Programs, Boston, personal communication, November 10, 1994). These organizations also cite widespread and detrimental reductions in resources for psychosocial services, particularly for inmates with HIV disease. Budget cuts often hit psychosocial and support services particularly hard. It is increasingly common for medical care and related services for inmates to be contracted out; this sometimes results in cutbacks in individual counseling, support groups, and other psychosocial services.

Eighty percent of state/federal systems report that correctional medical staff or public health personnel provide at least some HIV counseling. Nevertheless, the fact that so few survey responses described in detail a well-organized psychosocial support program is reason to be skeptical that these services are adequate. The number of correctional systems with full-time specialized counselors serving HIV-infected inmates is still low.

The availability of specialized professional staff to provide psychosocial and support services is low, and the availability of peer counselors remains very low as well. Table 5.6 shows that only sixteen state/federal systems (31 percent) and three city/county systems (10 percent) reported having HIV peer counselors. While lack of professional credentials and restrictions on inmate activities have been cited as obstacles for peer counseling programs in prison, this area merits a closer look. It may represent a cost-effective method of dealing with caseloads. Moreover, a wealth of creativity, resources, and commitment is often found in peer counselors. Research evidence suggests that peer counselors working in community-based outpatient drug treatment and HIV outreach programs, when given proper training and supervision, have been effective not only at counseling but also at developing creative interventions, as well as maintaining long-term participation (Abt Associates, 1995).

Support groups represent another important part of psy-

Table 5.6. Supportive Services for Inmates with HIV/AIDS, 1994.

Services Provided	U.S. State/Federal Prison Systems (n = 51)		U.S. City/County Jail Systems (n = 29)	
	n	%	n	%
Basic HIV information	48	94	23	79
HIV peer counselors available	16	31	3	10
Inmate peer-led support groups	20	39	3	11
Staff-led support groups	34	67	6	22
Support groups led by outside organizations	28	56	12	43

Source: NIJ/CDC questionnaire responses.

chosocial services to inmates with HIV/AIDS. HIV support groups conducted by correctional staff are reportedly offered in 67 percent of state/federal systems and 22 percent of responding city/county systems; peer-led support groups are reported by 39 percent of state/federal systems and 11 percent of responding city/county systems. Finally, 56 percent of state/federal systems and 43 percent of responding city/county systems offer HIV support groups led by outside organizations. Validation study results suggest that many individual facilities fail to provide the support groups reported as policy by the central offices of their systems. One-half to two-thirds of facilities in systems reportedly providing support groups said that they did not in fact offer such groups.

Examination of requests for technical assistance adds further weight to the perception that there is a need to improve the availability, diversity, and quality of psychosocial and supportive services for inmates with HIV disease. About one-third of the systems responding to the survey indicated an interest in technical assistance on HIV counseling.

Ongoing supportive services are particularly important to prisoners with HIV disease (and other serious illnesses) who may be experiencing serious psychological difficulties associated with their condition and high levels of stress related to dealing with such illness in a correctional setting. Stress can be particularly devastating for patients with HIV disease. A large body of research points to illness-related stress as having a major negative impact on the immune system (for example, Chesney & Folkman, 1994). Arguably, strategies to help inmates with HIV disease cope with their illness might be as important as access to therapeutic and prophylactic drugs. While psychosocial and supportive services are proven tools for helping people with stress, survey responses suggest they are far from well established in prisons and jails. Despite the low cost and standardization of stress-management programs, very few correctional systems reported having such programs.

"Buddy" programs have been developed by AIDS service organizations in the outside community to provide support for persons living with AIDS. A similar approach holds promise for inmates with AIDS. Buddy programs for inmates with AIDS are being developed in Massachusetts prisons and by the inmate peer program in the Oregon State Penitentiary.

If they cannot be released to die in the community, prisoners in the terminal stages of AIDS or other diseases may benefit from the availability of hospice care within correctional facilities. This is now offered in the Florida state system, and others, including New York, are considering it.

Drug Treatment

The dramatic increase in correctional populations during the past twelve years has been fueled by mass incarceration of drug users. At least some incarcerated drug users find ways to continue their drug use behind bars. Increasingly stringent mandatory sentencing provisions and persistently serious levels of substance abuse in the community will likely sustain the increase of the correctional population in general and of the number of drug-involved inmates in particular (U.S. General Accounting Office, 1991). In this context, provision of effective drug treatment remains both a challenge and an opportunity for correctional systems. As in the case of HIV education and prevention, correctional systems have ongoing access to large numbers of individuals in need of treatment. By providing effective treatment, they could help reduce relapse and recidivism rates. As the drug-using population increases, however, the resources needed for drug treatment, psychosocial, and medical services will also continue to increase.

Based on survey responses from thirty-four state/federal systems, a median of 70 percent of male inmates were estimated to have histories of drug use other than marijuana. Based on responses from thirty-two state/federal systems, a median of 71 percent of female inmates had histories of drug use other than marijuana. Among seventeen city/county systems, a median of 80 percent of male and female inmates were estimated to have used drugs other than marijuana.

Although various drug treatment modalities may be found in correctional settings, the 1994 survey requested information on only two: residential (separately housed within the correctional institution) treatment and ambulatory counseling. Responses to the 1994 NIJ/CDC survey reveal that more than forty-eight thousand inmates are participating either in residential treatment or ambulatory counseling in 37 state/federal systems. This figure represents only 5 percent of the total reported incarcerated populations of these systems, very low given the estimated prevalence of preincarceration drug use among inmates.

About 5,800 city/county inmates in sixteen systems were reported to be in residential or ambulatory treatment. This represents 4 percent of the inmate populations of these systems. The low percentage in jail systems is partly a result of short lengths of stay in such facilities. These figures suggest a continuing serious shortfall in drug treatment services in correctional facilities. On the other hand, it is clear that some correctional systems offer access to high-quality drug treatment. Information on the methods utilized by these systems to provide quality drug treatment may be useful so that they can be replicated elsewhere. In general, more systematic communication and sharing of strategies and modalities of substance abuse treatment would be useful.

Discharge Planning and Post-Release Services

There may be a temptation on the part of correctional authorities to reduce their medical services costs by seeking the release of inmates with AIDS and other illnesses. Regardless of how or when inmates with HIV/AIDS are released from prisons and jails, however, it is essential that comprehensive discharge planning be done so that inmates are connected with services they need in the community.

Eighty-two percent of state/federal systems and 55 percent of responding city/county systems reported providing discharge planning for inmates with HIV/AIDS. Table 5.7 shows the services reportedly offered by correctional systems as part of the discharge planning process. Between 49 and 71 percent of state/federal systems report making referrals, depending on the category of service, while only 16–25 percent of systems report making actual appointments for releases to obtain these services. Percentages are lower for both discharge planning referrals and arrangement of appointments in city/county systems. The more extensive the prerelease planning and arrangements, the greater the likelihood of follow-through by releases.

Table 5.7. Discharge Planning Services, 1994.

	U.S. State/Federal Prison Systems (n = 51)				U.S. City/County Jail Systems (n = 29)			
	Referral Made		Appointment Made		Referral Made		Appointment Made	
Services	n	%	n	%	n	%	n	%
Medicaid/related benefits	36	71	13	25	13	45	4	14
CD4 monitoring	33	65	12	24	13	45	4	14
Therapeutic medications	35	69	12	24	14	48	6	21
Substance abuse treatment	25	49	7	14	14	48	6	21
Ongoing HIV counseling	35	69	9	18	14	48	5	17
Psychosocial support	32	63	8	16	14	48	4	14

Source: NIJ/CDC questionnaire responses.

Actual facility-level performance may have even more short-comings than indicated by reported system-level policies. The validation study reveals that 62 percent of facilities in systems with policies to provide discharge planning reported actually providing such services. More than one-third of these facilities reported not providing discharge planning despite their central office's policy that it be done. A New York inmate stated that discharge planning was not occurring in some facilities despite a systemwide policy that facility parole officers help inmates with HIV/AIDS secure their benefits for medications (AIDS Drug Assistance Programs [ADAPs]) and Supplemental Security Income (SSI) prior to release. However, the inmate reported significant recent progress in discharge planning at his facility, especially for those inmates involved in an HIV support group led by the Catholic chaplain (anonymous inmate, personal communication, November 14, 1994).

A number of correctional systems have initiated special, and in some cases quite innovative, programs to improve discharge planning for inmates with HIV/AIDS. The Health Resources and Services Administration (HRSA) has funded a number of these programs under the Special Projects of National Significance (SPNS) component of the Ryan White Care Act. These programs seek not only to improve the process of discharge planning before inmates are released but also to improve follow-through and continuity of care once they return to the community. Examples of these programs are provided below. A key to success in many of these programs is collaboration among correctional systems, academic institutions, and medical centers in the community. The most successful programs also appear to be those that do not limit their assistance to medical treatment but rather attempt to address the full range of human and social service program needs of the client. These may include housing, employment training and placement, drug treatment, and other services. In general, the more the person being released can be helped to make the transition to life in the community, the less chance he or she will commit further crimes and return to prison.

Rhode Island

Rhode Island's discharge planning program involves the correctional department, Miriam Hospital, and Brown University. The program is staffed by part-time nurses who seek to provide full evaluation and discharge planning services for all HIV-infected inmates beginning at least three months prior to their discharge. The program also monitors and follows up on individuals' status and progress once they leave prison. In its first year of operation, the program provided services to 68 percent of HIV-infected inmates at the Rhode Island Adult Correctional Institution. Most of those inmates not reached had very short sentences (Dixon et al., 1993)

The prerelease evaluation in Rhode Island includes needs assessment and arrangements for medical care, substance abuse treatment, finances, housing, family support, child care, and employment. The discharge planning staff have established an extensive network of organizations in the community willing to provide services to releases. Under an arrangement with Miriam Hospital and Brown University, it is often possible for these releasees to be cared for by the same physicians who treated them in prison. Housing and substance-abuse services have posed particular challenges, but the program has established important linkages with a range of residential and outpatient treatment agencies as well as with housing services. Sunrise House is a particularly important linkage, providing long-term housing and supportive services for releasees with HIV and without families or others with whom they could live (Flanigan et al., 1995).

An indication of the effectiveness of the Rhode Island program comes from a comparison of short-term recidivism rates for participants and nonparticipants. Among women with HIV infection, 12 percent who had received discharge planning services returned to prison within six months, while 27 percent of those who had not participated in the program were back in prison within six months (Flanigan et al., 1996).

Maryland

In Maryland, medical case management is provided for inmates with HIV/AIDS beginning three to six months before their release. Through this process, inmates are qualified for Medicaid, SSI, and other benefits before they return to the community. The case management staff prepare and submit necessary paperwork while the inmate is still incarcerated. Moreover, the Maryland program has used the U.S. Department of Housing and Urban Development's Housing for People with AIDS (HPWA) program to locate subsidized housing for a number of releases. Housing is often a particularly difficult problem for inmates with HIV/AIDS returning to the community, many of whom do not have families willing to take them in (Boyle & Kummer, 1994).

A new program in Maryland, supported by CDC funds, is providing HIV prevention case management to inmates nearing release from selected state prisons. This involves intensive, individualized support and prevention counseling for inmates who are experiencing or are likely to experience difficulty initiating or sustaining positive behavioral change. In addition, case managers provide referrals for psychosocial and health service needs, such as housing, drug treatment, and medical and social services.

Connecticut

In collaboration with Yale University Medical School, the Connecticut correctional system has instituted a range of new programs for inmates with HIV/AIDS. One program seeks to improve discharge planning and follow-up for female HIV-infected inmates at Niantic who are returning to the New Haven area (Altice, 1994).

Investigation of barriers to follow-up on referrals revealed problems with long waiting lists for methadone maintenance and other substance-abuse treatment, and delayed eligibility for Medicaid and other benefits, as well as releasees' reluctance to contact agencies in the community unless they had been personally introduced to them prior to release. The Interfaith AIDS Network has received a contract to conduct discharge planning and follow-up for women inmates with HIV/AIDS about to be released to New Haven. A case manager from Interfaith AIDS Network visits Niantic several times each week to meet with inmates scheduled for release. The case manager works with the inmates to expedite the process of qualification for Medicaid and other benefits, to make appointments for medical treatment on the outside, and to find resources for substance abuse treatment, if appropriate. The case manager then follows up with inmates after they are released to ensure that they make appointments.

Among women involved with the program, rates of keeping appointments and following through on referrals have been quite high. Ninety-eight percent of the women kept initial medical appointments, and 77 percent were still under regular medical treatment six months after their release. Rates of successfully accessing methadone maintenance and some other services were not as high, but the program has clearly helped many HIV-infected women to obtain better support and care in the community.

Federal Bureau of Prisons

At its Lexington, Kentucky, medical facility for women, the Federal Bureau of Prisons has undertaken a broad collaborative program with the University of Kentucky Medical Center and the national network of AIDS Education and Training Centers (AETCs) funded by the U.S. Public Health Service. Using this network, female inmates with HIV/AIDS who are nearing release from Lexington are linked with medical providers in the communities to which they will return. The AETCs refer releases to providers in these communities. The prison medical staff then communicate with the providers to ensure continuity of treatment and care. In some instances, referral providers have been able to enroll releases in experimental treatment protocols (Macher, 1994).

Cook County (Chicago), Illinois

Discharge planning may be even more challenging in city/county jails, where lengths of stay are generally short and turnover rates are high. However, several large jail systems have undertaken efforts in this area. In Cook County, Illinois, case managers from Cermak Health Services meet with inmates and make referrals. Because of caseload size and short stays, referrals are often made after the inmate is released. Necessary medical records on the inmate are then forwarded to the referral provider. Case managers also work to contact releases who received HIV antibody tests in jail but were not informed of their results prior to their release (Howleit & Stauffer, 1994).

Self-Help Materials

Discharge planning for inmates with HIV/AIDS is lacking or inadequate in many correctional facilities. Moreover, even where prerelease planning is adequate, there may be insufficient support and follow-up once inmates return to the community. To address this need, the AIDS in Prison Project of the Osborne Association in New York City has provided some simple written guidance and offers ongoing assistance and support for former inmates with HIV/AIDS. The written guidance suggests prerelease steps (for example, arranging housing, obtaining necessary identification papers, applying for medical and other benefits, and accessing support and case management services) and provides specific information on organizations and resources that can help inmates make these arrangements. The guidelines also outline first steps for former inmates to take once they are released: report to your parole officer, find a case manager, maintain sobriety, and remain calm and be assured "that things will work out with patience and persistence" (Machon, Lopez, & Meletiche, 1994).

Chapter Six

A Report from the Frontline

Four Case Studies

Research on HIV/AIDS education programs at correctional institutions is a relatively new and important field of investigation. It is well known that the prevalence of HIV seropositive people is much higher in prisons than in the general population (Vlahov et al., 1991; Weisfuse et al., 1991; Dixon et al., 1993). As was pointed out in previous chapters, public health workers have realized that because of the concentration of HIV-seropositive individuals and injection drug users in prisons, correctional institutions provide an opportune place to address the public health needs of hard-to-reach populations (Glaser & Greifinger, 1993).

One such need is HIV/AIDS education. HIV/AIDS education within correctional institutions has the potential of reducing HIV transmission within prisons and decreasing the spread of infection in the general population through influencing the behavior of social offenders before they are released. The main goal of this study is to assist in the formation of HIV/AIDS risk-reduction educational programs by employing the inmates' perspectives in such programs. We assessed educational needs by examining behavioral risk factors before and during incarceration. We used exploratory research employing qualitative and quantitative analysis of inmate interview data and formal focus groups to determine subpopulations that could be targeted for education on particular risk factors.

This investigation is based on research at four different types of correctional institutions:

1. A state medical facility for adult males
2. An inner-city juvenile detention facility
3. A county jail for adults
4. A rural boot-camp-style prison for young males

The data was collected through interviews and focus groups. The number of inmates interviewed and the number of focus groups conducted at each site was as follows:

1. Twenty-nine interviews and one focus group at the state medical facility
2. Thirty male and seventeen female interviews and two male and two female focus groups at the inner-city juvenile detention facility
3. Twenty-five interviews and two focus groups with female inmates at the county jail
4. Twenty-five interviews and one focus group at the boot camp prison

A total of 126 inmates were interviewed and eight focus groups were conducted. After examining each penal institution separately, we discuss common themes and ramifications for policy.

The social offenders were told that the interviews and focus groups were to provide information for needs assessment, current program evaluation, and future program development. Each inmate was interviewed individually and was asked almost one hundred questions. The questionnaire covered demographic information, support systems, HIV/AIDS-related knowledge, attitudes and behavior, assessment of the current educational program, and recommendations for program development. The focus groups served to clarify, validate, and supplement responses in the personal interviews and revealed group perceptions of both HIV infection risk and educational programs. The focus groups consisted of at most twelve inmates drawn from those interviewed; the groups

lasted approximately ninety minutes. Evaluation of existing programs and recommendations for program development in regards
to an HIV/AIDS curriculum were the main questions addressed
during the focus groups. The social offenders were encouraged to
describe how to develop a program which would make them and
others continually practice safer sex and eliminate blood-contact
behaviors. Themes relevant to specific sites were also raised during the focus groups, such as drugs and sex within prison at the
adult male medical facility, the possible role of parents in
HIV/AIDS education at the youth detention facility, and issues
related to female prostitution at the county jail. The following depictions incorporate the findings from the inmate interviews
and the results of the focus groups at each of the four correctional
settings.

Adult Male Medical Facility

A West Coast medium-to-maximum-security state medical facility
for adult males was examined. The inmates have either physical or
mental health disabilities. This facility has a population of approximately 3,200 inmates with an average age of thirty-seven. The
racial and ethnic composition of the social offenders is approximately 37 percent black, 38 percent white, 20 percent Hispanic, 4
percent Asian, and 1 percent "other." Sentences range from one
year to life. Of the 3,100 inmates, about 470 (15 percent) are HIV
seropositive. These inmates are segregated in the evening but are
integrated with the general prison population during the day.

Key participant interviews were conducted among a random
sample of twenty-nine inmates from the adult male medical facility. The participants' ages ranged from nineteen to fifty-eight.
Eleven identified themselves as black, ten as white, seven as Hispanic, none as Asian, and one as "other." Almost 80 percent were
high school graduates, and 10 percent of the total sample had
completed college. Six of them reported that they were currently
married. About two-thirds had been convicted of violent crimes;
the length of sentence varied from one to 28.5 years.

As other studies have found (Brewer & Derrickson, 1992;
DiClemente et al., 1991) the social offenders had a high rate of

involvement in high-risk sex behaviors. All of them report having been sexually active. Forty-eight percent stated that they had had their first sexual encounter by age twelve, 82 percent by age sixteen, and 100 percent by age twenty-one. Four of the twenty-nine reported to have been forced to have sex at some time. In the three months before their incarceration, twelve (41 percent) said they had more than one partner, five (17 percent) social offenders said they had four or more, and one (3 percent) said he had thirty. Four of the twenty-nine inmates reported having male partners, while the one with thirty partners reported that they were all male. Eight (28 percent) said that they usually have anal sex. Seven (24 percent) reported having sex while in jail. Since conjugal visits are permitted for some inmates, this may explain the sexual activity while incarcerated, but in the focus group it was reported that some "promiscuous sex" takes place among the inmates. The inmates complained about a lack of access to condoms in prison but acknowledged that sexual activity does take place within the facility. One inmate complained about HIV/AIDS education being provided but not condoms: "But I am incarcerated so I can't go out and practice safe sex, so what are you doing for that individual? So why are you coming at me with just conversation?"

The social offenders also reported not consistently using condoms during sexual encounters prior to incarceration. Eighteen (62 percent) said that they never or almost never use a condom with their main sex partner. Of the twenty-two (76 percent) who stated that they had sex with someone other than their main sex partner, sixteen (55 percent) reported that they never or almost never used a condom with their other sex partners. When asked if they ever traded sex for something, eight (28 percent) answered in the affirmative.

The inmates also exhibited high-risk behavior for the transmission of HIV through sharing of needles and, to a lesser degree, by becoming a "blood brother." Just over a third of the inmates reported that they had injected drugs with a syringe; of those ten, all but one reported sharing needles. In the focus group it was stated that social offenders do find access to drugs and inject while in prison and that it is difficult to obtain a needle and bleach. Thus lack of such access could be indirectly promoting HIV transmission in the prison. As one inmate described the situation: "Some-how they should not have to get the death sentence just because they have the habit."

In the focus group, it became evident that many social offenders were repeatedly tattooed and had other blood-to-blood contact while incarcerated. Eighteen of the twenty-nine social offenders in the survey reported being tattooed either before or during incarceration, with thirteen of them using homemade equipment. (The prison has a new policy that makes tattooing illegal in the facility.) The social offenders said that people continue to tattoo using the same needles without bleach to wash them. Only three of the twenty-nine social offenders reported that they had had blood-to-blood contact with someone else by being made a blood brother.

In March 1993 an HIV/AIDS education and prevention program for all new inmates was started by a social worker, as part of the intake process. It provides approximately seven hundred new inmates per month with 30–60 minutes of education on HIV/AIDS prevention. The information is presented through a multimedia approach, including lecture, storytelling, inmate-developed skits, and video presentations. The teachers are from a pool of ten multiethnic peer educators. The two main goals of the curriculum are to teach the inmates how to reduce and eliminate the transmission of HIV/STD and to encourage compassion for those with HIV/AIDS.

In the survey, inmates were questioned about the current HIV/STD education program. Twenty-seven of twenty-nine said that they voluntarily attended the classes while incarcerated in this institution. They reported that the peer instructors made them feel comfortable and that they felt that the instructors were concerned about their health. The inmates also found the program helpful and said they learned something new each time they attended.

In the focus group, part of the discussion was centered around what type of educational program would lead people to behavior that would reduce their risk of being infected with HIV. The social offenders thought that fear combined with knowledge of how to avoid infection would cause some people to practice safer behaviors. They stated that the most effective educators would be people who are HIV-seropositive. The inmates also preferred a multiracial group of teachers so that everyone had an instructor of his race with whom he could identify. In the survey the social offenders overwhelmingly stated that the program should be repeated and consist of both one-on-one and group sessions.

During the focus group the inmates expressed pessimism over whether HIV education could stop everyone from practicing unsafe behaviors. They felt that some people "just don't care" and would continue to engage in high-risk behaviors. For example, they believed that some men had "weak minds" and would have sex when the opportunity arose without regard to the risks. Inmates also felt that some HIV seropositive individuals were not concerned with spreading the infection and in fact might even intend to do so. They cited HIV-seropositive inmates' sexually propositioning HIV-seronegative social offenders. The inmates also felt that it was unlikely that an HIV-seropositive social offender would pull out a separate needle if he had one while injecting drugs with a group because he would be afraid that he might be denied access to the drugs.

Inner-City Juvenile Detention Facility

The focus now shifts to an inner-city juvenile detention center on the West Coast. Approximately 25,000 youths enter this facility annually. At any one time, about 1,800 youth are in the standard detention facility, for an average stay of two to three weeks; an additional 1,800 are in a residential treatment camp facility for an average stay of six months. The offenders, of whom 90 percent are male, range in age from nine to eighteen with an average age of 15.5. Their average reading level is at the fifth grade. The racial and ethnic composition of the inmates is approximately 55 percent Hispanic, 35 percent black, 9.5 percent white, and 0.5 percent Asian. Sixty percent are repeat offenders.

Thirty males and seventeen females were randomly selected for interviews from the male and female facilities' populations. The males ranged in age from twelve to nineteen, the females from fourteen to eighteen; the mean ages were 16.2 and 15.5, respectively. The racial and ethnic breakdown for both sexes combined was twenty (43 percent) Hispanics, seventeen (36 percent) blacks, five (11 percent) whites, four (9 percent) Asians, and one (2 percent) "other." One male was currently married, and one male and one female were separated. All but three males among the interviewees claimed English as their primary language, one reported Spanish, and two reported other languages. Only three of the forty-seven interviewees had graduated from high school, with mean years of schooling equal to 9.4. Just over half had been arrested once before. The length of the current sentences averaged twenty-one months. Eleven (37 percent) of the males and six (35 percent) of the females had been convicted of violent offenses. Besides conducting the survey, we held four focus groups at this facility (two male and two female groups).

The inmates reported becoming sexually active at very early ages. All of the females and all but four of the males reported having had sex. The mean age of first sexual encounter was thirteen for the females and twelve for the males. Two of the males reported that their first sexual encounter was at six, while others reported ages seven, eight, nine, and ten. Three of the males and seven of the females reported having been forced to have sex at some time in their lives. The low reported ages of the males' first sexual encounter is questionable because of the uncertain validity of the males' answers to the question given varying definitions perceived for "sex for the first time."

The male focus groups at times lacked seriousness, joked, and talked on tangents; some participants dwelled on discussions of sex (requiring the facilitator to redirect the discussion). In one of the male groups, some of the inmates admitted that they were not listening to the facilitator. The inmate who broached the topic said it was because a court appearance set for the next day was occupying his mind. Others said that they did not pay attention because they did not care. When pressed by the facilitator to explain why they did not care, the inmates explained that they did not care because the facilitator did not care about them (tension existed in this group between the facilitator and the inmates). Two problems specific to young males were the questionable veracity of their survey responses and a lack of seriousness during the focus groups. Working with young males in prison presents special concerns because of immaturity. Many of them have developed tough attitudes as a defense mechanism to survive gang and street life.

The inmates were asked about their sexual activity and condom use to determine their level of high-risk behavior. The males reported having had between zero and eleven partners (with a mean of 3.6) in the three months prior to incarceration. The females had fewer partners in general, with a range of zero to three partners with an outlier of eight (mean 1.4). None of the males reported having had sex with a male, but one of the females said she had had sex with two female partners in the three months before incarceration. Combining both sexes, 65 percent said that they usually had vaginal sex, 28 percent oral sex, and 7 percent anal sex. One of the males and one of the females stated that they had traded sex for alcohol. Sexual activity while in prison was reported by two of the inmates.

These youths consistently failed to protect themselves with condoms during sexual encounters. Twelve (71 percent) of the seventeen females and fifteen (50 percent) of the thirty males reported that they have a main sex partner. Only three of the males and two of the females always use a condom with their main sex partner. Fourteen of the young men said that they "always" use a condom with someone other than their main sex partner, and eight stated that they "almost always" used one. Five of the females said that they "always" used one with someone other than their main partner, four reported "almost always" using one, and one said she "sometimes" used a condom.

During the focus groups some males stated repeatedly that if they did not have a condom available they would have sex anyway or that in the "heat of the moment" they would not think of using one. In both male and female focus groups, complaints were made that condoms reduce pleasure. One young woman said that she always practiced safe sex mainly because she had to live for her daughter. Another female avoids high-risk behavior because she wants to be a doctor and "because I have goals, dreams, aspirations, it's just something I have to do."

Drug and alcohol use increased the inmates' risk of infection. Four of the males reported using intravenous drugs, but only one said that he shared his needles. Results of the survey revealed that none of the females reported using intravenous drugs (possibly due to the sensitive nature of the question) but one admitted injection drug use during the focus group. Sixteen (53 percent) of the males and five (29 percent) of the females said that they had sex while drunk. Twenty-four (80 percent) of the males and fourteen

(82 percent) of the females used drugs to get "high." When asked if drinking alcohol or using drugs interferes with practicing safer sex, five of the males and five of the females said yes. One of the males stated he would not remember to use a condom after drinking because alcohol "impairs" his mind.

The inmates participated in activities other than sharing drug needles that led to blood contact. Proportionately more of the females (71 percent) reported having tattoos than males (47 percent). All of the participants knew that HIV could be transmitted through tattoo needles. Two males and one female reported having gotten homemade versus professional tattoos. Four of the males and two of the females said that they exchanged blood by becoming blood brothers or sisters with someone.

The attendees' evaluations of the current HIV/AIDS education program were positive. The current program of reproductive health education is a six-hour program, divided into one hour devoted to HIV/AIDS, two hours to STD, and three hours to sexuality and reproduction issues. The material is presented in a lecture by a health educator and a video. There is no one-on-one counseling. Twenty-six of the forty-seven youths reported attending the voluntary HIV/AIDS classes. Twenty-two of the twenty-six said it was helpful, and twenty said that they learned something new. In the focus group, one individual expressed the belief that HIV could be transmitted by saliva through kissing someone with a cold sore, or sharing a pipe. This misperception is an example of the finding of Zimmerman et al. (1991) among Pennsylvania inmates that a low level of knowledge is associated with an increased perception of risk of infection through casual contact. The misperception illustrates the need among inmates for basic HIV/AIDS transmission education.

Most of the focus group discussions focused on how to develop the most effective HIV/AIDS education program. The youths were quite specific about aspects of the curriculum and what type of person would make the most effective instructor. The most common theme was that people very sick with AIDS should be shown in person or in videos; the latter should have "really gross pictures." As one youth put it, "Like a movie . . . you look at it, you don't think about it because you don't have it, but if you look at somebody who has the disease and you're looking at it and you flip out, you say damn! I don't want to look like that. Got to look at the real thing."

The social offenders also said that the material should be informative about HIV/AIDS transmission. It should be presented on their level with vocabulary they can understand. Issues of concern to all sexual orientations should be covered. Videos should be about people they can relate to racially, ethnically, and socially. One youth said that when a story about a wealthy gay man with AIDS was presented, the youths laughed and thought him a "fool." The young men said that they found information about mothers with HIV boring, but the young women felt the contrary and wanted that sort of information included in a program. Both males and females said that they needed repeated exposure to an HIV/AIDS program for it to be effective. Pessimistically, it was stated repeatedly that whatever the program, after a course of about six months the lessons are forgotten. Both male and female youths felt that an HIV/AIDS program should be fun. They suggested the development of games, comic books, computer games, word puzzles, and video games to teach about HIV transmission. One interesting idea was to develop an HIV/AIDS museum for educational purposes.

Discussion also centered around what characteristics an effective HIV/AIDS instructor should have other than academic knowledge of the virus and disease. Echoing the discussion of curriculum, the youths preferred an instructor with AIDS. One person stated that an instructor with AIDS was more credible than a physician. From the social offenders' statements, it was not clear whether a person who was HIV-positive was acceptable or only a person with AIDS symptoms. The instructor should be someone they can identify with through similarities in age and life experience. Gang members would best be reached by gang members.

The idea of celebrity instructors came up a few times in the focus groups. Some said they would listen to Magic Johnson, while it was also expressed that maybe he was not really infected with HIV because he shows no symptoms of AIDS. One young woman said she would have listened to rap artist Easy-E if he had come to speak at the prison before he died because he got AIDS from heterosexual sex. Another said she would not listen to Easy-E but would listen to rhythm and blues singer Brandy if she came in and spoke with them about her life, because Brandy interests her. The tone was one of fantasizing that their music idols cared about them.

One theme that the young females clearly and repeatedly expressed in the focus groups was that they needed someone to care about them, and that this would make it easier for them to change their behavior. One inmate said that she had been sentenced to this facility five or six times, but that every time she told her mother and her mother's boyfriend that she would change, they had no faith in her and she failed. Another said that she never found anyone who cared about her or sacrificed their time to help her until she started attending Narcotics Anonymous in prison. Her mother had died from drugs and her father had encouraged her to commit crimes; he is now serving a twenty-five-years-to-life sentence. Some of the women said that the most effective HIV/AIDS educator would be someone who cares and who repeatedly comes back to make sure they are listening to him or her, someone who would even keep in touch with them after their release. One inmate said that she would follow a recommendation to be tested every six months for HIV infection if someone were there to remind and prod her; she interjected, "Even at home, if someone was on my back, I wouldn't be in trouble." An HIV/AIDS education program cannot fill the role of a functioning parent, but the need for repeated visits by a caring instructor seems important in reducing the high-risk behavior of the young female social offenders.

The young males lacked concern for their personal welfare. This was expressed in repeated statements that HIV transmission prevention education cannot reach everyone because some people just want to have sex and do not care about the consequences. After one such statement, the facilitator encouraged the inmate to explain why. The inmate replied, "Drugs, locked up, family problems." The facilitator prodded the inmate to detail the types of family problems; the inmate answered, "Nobody cares about you, nobody asks you how you're doing." Another negative attitude that an HIV/AIDS education program would have to overcome among some of the inmates is the idea that if AIDS does not kill you then a bullet on the street will, so why practice safer sex (the "you must die from something" syndrome)? In this vein, one young man said while discussing development of an educational program, "You're gonna die anyway . . . it's a joke, it's a joke to me." Hence it becomes obvious that HIV/AIDS education programs designed for young male inmates will need compassionate instructors to firmly encourage inmates to reduce high-risk behaviors.

Adult County Jail

This section focuses on women in an adult county jail in a major Midwestern city. The facility houses about 120 women with sentences averaging about three months. The inmates have been convicted of drug-related and sex-trading offenses. Approximately 65 percent of the women are black. When the survey of these inmates was conducted, no formal group HIV/AIDS education program was in place. Four staff members were certified by the state health department to provide HIV/AIDS education to the inmates, and plans were underway to begin a program.

The twenty-five inmates interviewed were randomly selected from the daily log of those who were arrested for prostitution, failed to make bail, and were sentenced to at least thirty days. Their ages ranged from nineteen to forty-nine, with an average age of thirty-two years. Eighteen identified themselves as black, five as white, and two as belonging to a nondescriptive "other" race group. Twenty-four of the twenty-five have English as their primary language, and one reported a language other than English or Spanish. Eleven graduated from high school; the average number of years of education was 11.4. Two of the women were married, fifteen were single, and eight were separated, divorced, or widowed. The sentences ranged from one month to one year, with twelve of the women having a one-month sentence. Two focus groups comprising eight women each were also conducted. During the focus groups the women were very cooperative and respectful of the facilitator, referring to her as "ma'am."

The average age of first sexual encounter for the women was fifteen. When asked how many partners they had had in the three months before entering prison, eleven reported having only one, seven said they had had between two and seven, and four stated that they had had seventy-five or more male partners. (The high figures seem reasonable for commercial sex workers.) They all reported having mainly vaginal or oral sex as opposed to anal sex. Fourteen said that they had a main sex partner, but only six used a condom with him. Sixteen said that they have sex with someone other than their main partner, but only eleven stated that they always used a condom with these partners.

The inmates discussed a number of ways in which prostitution increases the risk of HIV infection. Most of the women, twenty out of twenty-five, reported that they had traded sex, predominantly for money. The focus groups discussed the dangers of prostitution and the relationship to HIV/AIDS. Some women equated prostitution and AIDS and believed that you could not work as a street-level prostitute without exposing yourself to the risk of becoming infected with HIV. The women complained that working the streets is a violent occupation. They said, "Some prostitutes are murdered and others are raped." Rape exposes even prostitutes who insist that their clients use a condom to the possibility of becoming infected with the HIV virus. Sixteen (64 percent) of the inmates reported that they had been forced to have sex at some time. Besides rape, the women admitted that the average prostitute is not going to turn down a "date" who has fifty dollars in hand if they do not have a condom available. Seven of the women reported that clients would try to keep them from using a condom each time they had sex, but only one said that she would have sex with a partner or client who refused to use a condom. Drug usage also influences the ability of prostitutes to protect themselves from HIV/AIDS infection. During the focus group the point was made that if a prostitute is a drug addict and needs a fix, she is not going to care whether her client uses a condom, as long as she can get the money she needs to buy her drugs.

Drugs increased the risk of the women being infected with HIV in two ways: through sharing needles and interfering with their ability to practice safer sex. Twenty-three (92 percent) of the women reported using drugs to get high, but only six (24 percent) said that they had injected drugs. Of those six, four said that they had shared needles. Seventeen (68 percent) of the inmates reported having sex while drunk. Eight of the women said that when they were drunk or high they would not bother to try to protect themselves from being infected with HIV.

These inmates also participated in unsafe blood contact practices other than sharing drug needles. Four of the women had been tattooed; three had had it professionally done. Only two of the women believed that you could not contract the AIDS virus from the needles used for tattooing. Five (20 percent) of the women reported becoming a blood sister. This is slightly higher than the rate found among the male social offenders at other facilities in this study.

As stated above, these inmates were not exposed to any formal HIV/AIDS education program while incarcerated at this county jail. From statements made during the focus groups, one can readily see that a program is needed to teach basic HIV transmission education. Inmates believed that HIV infection could be transmitted by saliva, as in sharing a glass or a pipe with someone infected with HIV. It was also stated that mosquitoes and sexual relations with dogs could transmit the virus. These types of misperceptions again corroborate the finding by Zimmerman et al. (1991) that a lack of HIV/AIDS knowledge generally increases the perception of risk of transmission through casual contact. They also demonstrate the immediate need for HIV/AIDS education.

The inmates discussed what type of educational program they thought would be most effective in helping them eliminate their high risk of HIV transmission behavior. The women were very clear in stating that they wanted to see people who were very sick with AIDS. The curriculum should include pictures of people very sick and emaciated with AIDS. It should show the effects of the virus from "the first days to the last." The best instructor would be someone who is "about to die" or "almost dying from" AIDS. The person should also be knowledgeable and the type who wants to keep people from becoming infected, not someone who is angry and wants to spread it to everyone. The inmates believed that without seeing the deathly effects of the virus, they would not take the educational program or the disease seriously.

It should be noted that despite the harshness of these statements about needing to be educated by seeing the devastating effect of AIDS, in one of the focus groups compassion was expressed for people with AIDS. This may be partially because the participants were women and historically females have been seen to be more expressive and emotive than males. The only other focus group in which sympathy was expressed for people with AIDS was in one of the young women's focus groups in the inner-city juvenile detention facility.

Boot Camp Correctional Institution

The last site discussed is a boot-camp-style correctional institution in the rural South. Each month, approximately one hundred male youths aged 17–25 begin a three-month sentence in this facility. This alternative type of facility segregates the youths from the possible negative consequences of exposure to violent and older inmates. The racial composition of the facility is approximately 85 percent black and 15 percent white.

The participants in the study were randomly selected from a single group of entrants after they were exposed to a brief Red Cross HIV/AIDS education program. The ages of the twenty-five male inmates interviewed ranged from seventeen to twenty-three. Eighteen identified themselves racially as black, five as white, and two did not respond to that question. For all of them, English was their primary language. Four of the twenty-five were high school graduates, with the mean number of years of schooling completed equal to ten. One of the men was married, one was separated, and the rest were single. They were all serving a three-month sentence for a nonviolent offense. The size of the focus group was eleven inmates.

A number of the inmates were involved in high-risk sexual behavior for HIV transmission. All of the twenty-five young men reported having had sex, with fourteen years the mean age of the first sexual encounter. When asked how many sexual partners they had had in the last three months before they were incarcerated, thirteen said one, nine reported between two and five, one said twelve, and two stated they had had as many as twenty and twenty-five partners. The inmates reported having sex exclusively with females; most of them usually had vaginal sex. Twenty-one of the twenty-five said that they had a main sex partner. Fifteen said they never used a condom with their main sex partner. Sixteen of the twenty-five also reported that they had sex with someone other than their main sex partner. Fourteen reported that they always used a condom when having sex with someone other than their main partner.

Fourteen of the sixteen who had sex with someone other than their main sex partner reported always using a condom with the person other than their main partner. This high percentage (88 percent) seems to contradict the attitudes expressed during the focus group, where many of the statements condoned condom usage. Participants expressed that in the "heat of the moment" they just didn't think of protecting themselves through condom use even if they had one with them at the time. Complaints that using a condom is not as "passionate," "it does not feel good," and "it is like taking a shower with a raincoat" were voiced. Purchasing condoms was described as embarrassing and discouraging use. The comment was also made that "girls" want to have sex with you after you get them "high" but that the male loses his ability to think clearly after using alcohol and drugs and is less likely to use a condom. In the survey, eighteen of the twenty-five said that they had sex while drunk, but only two said that using alcohol or drugs prevented them from using condoms to protect themselves from contracting STD or HIV/AIDS.

This contradiction between relatively high reported condom usage in the survey and negative statements about condom usage in the focus groups brings up the issue of the veracity of the responses of the youth. In any survey, response bias is an issue (Sudman & Bradburn, 1974). It is possible that in the survey the inmates overstated their usage of condoms. During the focus group, probably due in a large measure to their age, at times the social offenders joked or clowned around, bragged, and responded in a manner to please the facilitator. For example, when discussing condoms, one inmate said in a nonchalant manner that he was not only going to always use a condom but "let's double up" and use two at a time. This along with other unrealistically positive statements may have been said to please the facilitator or to mock the research exercise. Standard research difficulties are exacerbated while working with confined youths because of age and situational factors. An example of a situational factor is that despite promises of anonymity, social offenders may think that their responses could affect their confinement conditions.

A small number of the inmates reported other possible high-risk sexual experiences. Three of the youths stated that they had traded sex for drugs or alcohol, and one said he had traded sex for money. Four reported that they had been forced to have sex at some time in their life. None reported having sex while in the boot camp facility. Because of the high level of supervision in this facility, that is not a surprising finding.

Only one of the inmates reported ever injecting drugs; he stated that he never shared his needle with anyone. Tattooing, another source of possible blood contact, showed a higher prevalence than drug injection, with twelve of the twenty-five reporting having gotten a tattoo and only three of those done professionally. Nineteen reported that they knew that tattooing could transmit the AIDS virus, but it could not be determined from the survey whether this knowledge was acquired before or after the tattooing took place. Three of the inmates also reported participating in the high-risk behavior of becoming blood brothers with someone else.

The current program for HIV/AIDS education is run by the Red Cross. The Red Cross curriculum covers the topics of risk reduction as related to drug use and sexual behavior, and it informs the social offenders about HIV testing as well. The class lasts for about ninety minutes, with a video and instruction by a Red Cross volunteer. The inmates are exposed to this HIV/AIDS risk-reduction class during both their first and last weeks of incarceration. The inmates' responses in the surveys rated the current program highly. They said the classes were helpful and educational. The social offenders also reported that the Red Cross health educator made them feel comfortable and showed concern for their health.

During the focus group, the inmates made three concrete suggestions on how to improve the current HIV/AIDS education program in the boot camp prison. First, they said that they would like more HIV/AIDS education. Relative to drug abuse education, they receive very little. They reported that two hours a day for six to eight days are devoted to drug education, but only a single ninety-minute session at the beginning of their sentences is spent on HIV/AIDS education. At some points, the inmates identified with the situations presented in the drug videos, but not as much with the HIV/AIDS video, perhaps because of the limited amount of material that could be presented with only one HIV/AIDS video. Second, they suggested that the videos should show people with AIDS suffering greatly from their illness and that this would make the social offenders take HIV risk-reduction more seriously. Finally, it was also similarly suggested that having program instructors as well as inviting guest speakers who are very sick with AIDS would make the social offenders take a more serious attitude to the prevention of HIV/AIDS transmission.

The social offenders in a number of focus groups again made statements of their belief that some people could never be reached by HIV/AIDS education and would always continue to partake of high-risk behavior. Twice it was stated that some people just do not care and would not use a condom even if they had one with them. One inmate made an analogy between smokers and people who do not use condoms: even though they know their behaviors put them at risk for fatal diseases they persist in their behavior. Another reason why they thought that HIV/AIDS education cannot reach everyone is that some people think—albeit irrationally—that they cannot become infected. It was also stated that some men would not turn down an opportunity to have sex even if a condom were not available. The most negative comment by one of the inmates was that HIV/AIDS education is important in prisons because some social offenders with HIV/AIDS do not care and will rape while in prison or after they are released without taking into consideration the possibility of transmitting the infection to their victims.

Targeting HIV/AIDS Education Programs

Two benefits of targeting HIV/AIDS education programs to specific groups are increased effectiveness and efficiency (Gillies & Carballo, 1990). Effectiveness is increased when material and its presentation are tailored to a group so that it is easily absorbed by the members. Factors such as cultural relevancy, vocabulary, and characteristics of an instructor are important in this regard. Targeting increases efficiency by allowing limited public health funds to be spent on programs directed at the highest risk groups. It is believed that the benefits of targeting in controlling the spread of HIV infection outweigh its possible negative effects: social stigmatization of targeted groups and promotion of a false sense of safety among the nontargeted population (Gillies & Carballo, 1990). In this section, we present the results of three multivariate logistic regressions which examine the relationship between high-risk behaviors and gender, race and ethnicity, age, and violent or non-violent offense. This exploratory analysis can be used as a foundation for research to target HIV/AIDS education programs.

The three dichotomous dependent variables of the multivariate regressions represent always using a condom when having sex with someone other than one's main sex partner, ever having injected drugs with a syringe, and ever having been tattooed. The first reflects high-risk behavior in regard to sexuality; the other two relate to the risks of HIV transmission associated with needle use. "Always" using a condom is coded as 1, with "not always" coded as 0; similarly, "ever" injecting drugs is coded as 1 and "never" as 0, and "ever" tattooed as 1 and "never" tattooed as 0.

Four dimensions were captured by the independent variables: gender, race/ethnicity, age, and conviction for a violent versus a nonviolent offense. All of these characteristics might be expected to have some effect on high-risk behavior. For some behaviors, women might be expected to have higher rates than men, such as prostitution (Smith et al., 1991). The generally higher rates of HIV prevalence in prison populations among minorities, women, and older inmates (Vlahov et al., 1991) also point to the possible significance of these dimensions. Violent offenders may be higher risk takers than nonviolent offenders. All of these characteristics have the potential of being used in targeting HIV/AIDS education programs. In the regressions, all but age (an interval-level variable) were coded as dummy variables. The four Asians and one person who identified himself racially as "other" were removed from the sample because of the small numbers in those categories, leaving black, white, and Hispanic as the three racial/ethnic groups analyzed.

The results of the three multivariate regressions are presented in Tables 6.1, 6.2, and 6.3. In the first regression, the dependent variable assessed whether one always used condoms when having sex with someone other than one's main partner. The only statistically significant variable was *age* ($p = .0349$). The coefficient estimate for *age* suggests that every additional year of age is worth a reduction in the odds of always using a condom with a partner other than one's main sex partner by a factor of 0.947. The second regression, reported in Table 6.2, has "ever injected drugs with a syringe" as the dependent variable. In this case the independent variables *black* ($p = 0.03$) and *age* ($p = .05$) are statistically signifi-

Table 6.1. Logistic Regression of *Always Using a Condom with Someone Other Than One's Main Sex Partner* **on** *Violent/Nonviolent Offense* **and Demographic Variables (***n* = 88**).**

	Coefficient	Odds Ratio	p
Sex	-0.3207	0.726	0.5360
Black	0.3128	1.367	0.6031
Hispanic	-0.2171	0.805	0.7761
Age	-0.0540	0.947	0.0349
Violent	-0.7735	0.461	0.1347
Intercept	1.573		0.1039
-2 Log likelihood	110.161		0.0436

Source: Braithwaite & Mayberry, 1996.

Table 6.2. Logistic Regression of *Ever Injected Drugs with a Syringe* **on** *Violent/Nonviolent Offense* **and Demographic Variables (***n* = 94**).**

	Coefficient	Odds Ratio	p
Sex	0.6979	2.010	0.3519
Black	-1.4844	0.227	0.0303
Hispanic	-1.0505	0.350	0.1966
Age	0.0528	1.054	0.0525
Violent	0.4024	1.495	0.5298
Intercept	-2.8267		0.0066
-2 Log likelihood	71.861		0.0162

Source: Braithwaite & Mayberry, 1996.

cant. The independent variable *black* reduces one's odds of using intravenous drugs while *being older* increases them. Finally, in the third model it is shown that blacks have significantly reduced odds of ever being tattooed compared to whites. It should be noted that the sample size varied in the regressions because of missing values.

Table 6.3. Logistic Regression of *Ever Been Tattooed* on *Violent/Nonviolent Offense* and Demographic Variables (*n* = 112).

	Coefficient	Odds Ratio	p
Sex	0.7475	2.112	0.0954
Black	-1.0959	0.334	0.0350
Hispanic	0.2361	1.226	0.7032
Age	-0.0216	0.979	0.3160
Violent	0.6202	0.538	0.1629
Intercept	0.6851		0.3877
-2 Log likelihood	141.129		0.0168

Source: Braithwaite & Mayberry, 1996.

These exploratory analyses raise some interesting issues. One is that HIV/AIDS education is necessary for inmates of all ages, not just for the younger social offenders. Indeed, HIV prevalence is higher among inmates over twenty-five years of age than among those younger than twenty-five for both sexes (Vlahov et al., 1991). Considering that HIV prevalence in prisons is higher for blacks than for whites, it seems surprising that incarcerated blacks are less likely to have engaged in the high-risk behaviors of injection drugs and tattooing than whites, controlling for age, gender, and violence of the offense (Vlahov et al., 1991). One possible explanation may be that people in rural areas participate less in intravenous drug activities and tattooing than those in urban areas. Our sample may have a higher concentration of rural blacks than of rural whites. The survey did not ask if one lived in an urban or rural area, and therefore such a variable was not included in the regression models. The most reasonable conclusion that can be drawn from the logistic regression analysis is that one should not solely target younger inmates for HIV/AIDS education, because the older population is also active in high-risk behaviors.

Conclusion

The input from social offenders at four sites through surveys and focus groups was very helpful in generating valuable recommendations for HIV/AIDS education program development. The most often repeated inmate recommendation from all of the correctional institutions was to have videos showing people, or visitors, who are very sick with AIDS. They said that this is what is necessary for them to take HIV risk-reduction education seriously. Seeing the long-term consequences of HIV infection would grab their attention, frighten them, and motivate them to change. Of course, this must be done realistically, without exaggerating the dangers and thereby causing greater fear as with some antidrug films of the 1960s and early 1970s. To create such videos and to find and present such visitors would be challenging. All of this should be done while preserving the dignity of the sick, avoiding all traces of exploitation, and without stigmatizing those suffering from AIDS.

Other recommendations can also be drawn from the data in regard to curriculum development. The material presented should be sound in terms of presenting the basic facts about HIV/AIDS and HIV transmission. It should be presented in a culturally relevant manner so that the inmates can identify with the examples. Vocabulary must be on a level equivalent to the audience. Exposure to the information must be repeated to make a lasting impression. The younger inmates at the inner-city juvenile facility and at the boot camp think that information should be presented in a "fun" manner by developing computer and video games, word puzzles, and comic books which teach about HIV transmission. The females asked for information relating motherhood to HIV/AIDS, whereas young males stated specifically that the same material would bore them and turn them off. Another important recommendation which can be drawn from the input of the inmates is that combining a program on violence reduction with HIV/AIDS education for inner-city youths involved in gangs may be helpful in providing the hope for a future and therefore motivation to reduce behaviors with high risk for HIV transmission.

The inmates also presented valuable insights into the characteristics of an effective HIV/AIDS education instructor. An HIV-infected health educator, preferably already showing AIDS symptoms, would be the most trusted and effective instructor. Inmates would pay the most attention to instructors with whom they can identify racially, ethnically, and in terms of social origins and experience. This calls for racial and ethnic diversity in both HIV/AIDS health educators and characters in educational material. The social offenders also want an instructor who cares about them and their health; this was especially true for the young women at the inner-city juvenile facility. One way in which this feeling can be fostered is by having repeated visits by the same health educators.

The findings of the multivariate logistic regression suggest that all inmates must be educated about HIV/AIDS. They show that the older inmates are probably more active in high-risk behaviors than the younger ones. Yet the educational needs of young inmates cannot be ignored because they too are active in behaviors with high risk for HIV transmission (DiClemente et al., 1991). At two sites, the county jail for female adults and the inner-city juvenile detention facility, some inmates had never been exposed to HIV/AIDS education. These social offenders expressed erroneous beliefs about HIV transmission. There is a need to reach all inmates, through either mandatory classes or the development of interesting programs which attract all inmates voluntarily. Even in prisons with relatively low rates of HIV infection, universal education is important (Andrus et al., 1989).

Much has been written about the prevalence of sex and drug use in prisons and the consequent need, from a public health perspective, for condoms and clean needles to be made available to inmates (Harding, 1987; Pagliaro & Pagliaro, 1992; Brewer & Derrickson, 1992). This investigation also found that social offenders engage in high-risk behaviors such as unprotected sex, intravenous drug use, and tattooing while incarcerated. This was especially true of the adult male medical facility, where 24 percent of the inmates reported having sex in prison. In that facility, inmates in the focus group complained about the difficulty of obtaining condoms, clean needles, and bleach. These findings reinforce the belief that more must be done to realistically face the challenges of HIV transmission within correctional facilities. The recommendations developed in this study for HIV/AIDS education in prisons will be helpful in combating these problems, but the lessons learned cannot be applied in correctional institutions without access to condoms and clean needles.

Chapter Seven

Prison Personnel
Gatekeepers to Education and Prevention

Attitudes about HIV/AIDS may have important consequences for social behavior when HIV-seropositive and HIV-seronegative individuals are brought together in a closed environment, specifically a prison. The issue of HIV/AIDS in prisons has been the subject of considerable debate (McKee, Markova, & Power, 1995). Pagliaro and Pagliaro (1992) emphasized the importance of obtaining unbiased and factually correct information concerning HIV and AIDS knowledge among inmates and staff. Remarkably little research has attempted to systematically determine prison staff knowledge about and attitudes towards HIV/AIDS issues. Most of the research focuses on inmates' perspectives of HIV/AIDS infection. This chapter reports survey results of perceptions of correctional staff ($n = 65$) relative to HIV/AIDS issues.

Even though occupational exposure is rare, fear of HIV transmission from inmates is commonplace among corrections personnel. A majority of the Illinois probation and detention workers revealed that they would feel at least somewhat uncomfortable supervising a confirmed or suspected HIV-antibody-positive offender; and there are examples of correctional officers declining to perform their duties for fear of contracting HIV (Lurigio, Petraitis, & Johnson, 1991). Their attitudes towards HIV will directly affect the way they treat HIV-positive inmates, educational programs offered to inmates, and related public health issues. Personnel deserve more attention in the study of prison HIV epidemics.

Having detailed information about HIV enhances educational programs for inmates and prison staff. More-informed prison officers can become HIV educators as well as client advocates, contributing much more to public health in preventing the spread of HIV. One main goal of this survey of correctional staff is to explore personnel attitudes regarding HIV/STDs risk factors among inmates as well as their evaluation of the HIV/AIDS risk-reduction programs in correctional institutions.

Staff Attitudes Toward HIV/AIDS

Given the high number of HIV-positive inmates reported in Chapter One, negative attitudes toward people with AIDS may be especially problematic in correctional facilities. With the already high incidence of AIDS and no apparent cure in sight, prison officials must deal with fear of HIV transmission and with discrimination against those having or suspected of having AIDS (Mahaffey & Marcus, 1995). When negative attitudes toward HIV-seropositive inmates are apparent on the part of correctional staffers, serious management problems can be anticipated. For example, countries such as Germany, Belgium, France, and the United States have experienced serious disruptions in penal establishments because of panic reactions to HIV/AIDS among inmates and prison staff (McKee et al., 1995). Also, National Institute of Justice (NIJ) reports have consistently indicated that correctional officers fear being infected with HIV while at work (Mahaffey & Marcus, 1995). Previous studies showed that homophobia, knowledge about AIDS, and intolerant attitudes about AIDS are related. People who are more homophobic are less knowledgeable about AIDS, report negative attitudes toward people with AIDS, and are more fearful of getting HIV through casual transmission.

Correctional officers often point to the intimate nature of their contact with inmates as justification for their fears. Officers may be especially concerned about the risk of HIV infection from being bitten, spit upon, or stuck with sharp objects, or from coming into contact with inmates' urine, feces, or blood (Mahaffey & Marcus, 1995). These fears may interfere with correctional officers' efficiency and ability to do their jobs. Although the panic over AIDS contagion, which led to threats of staff walkouts and inmate riots in the mid-1980s, has abated, the contagion hypothesis persists. Such fear has fueled demands from staff unions for mandatory antibody testing and segregation of all HIV-positive inmates, and it has contributed to negligent treatment of HIV-positive inmates by correctional staff. Fear of AIDS contagion among officers may even influence the health care of HIV-infected inmates, as correctional officers are often the link between inmates and health care providers.

In what may be the first published study dealing specifically with correctional officers and AIDS, Kamerman (1991) examined the attitudes of thirteen correctional officers who worked with AIDS patients. Some of the officers indicated that they felt more secure working with AIDS-diagnosed inmates compared to working in the general population. Most of the officers stated that participating in prison AIDS education programs and seeing other officers working with AIDS patients helped to reduce their fears of contracting the disease.

McKee et al. (1995) studied 480 male inmates and 500 male staff from seven Scottish prisons to ascertain perception of risk and attitudes towards HIV/AIDS. The research did not focus on the staff's perceptions of inmate risk. Nevertheless, their research revealed some important aspects of the attitudes within the prison settings. Their findings suggest that prison staff perceive prison as a higher-risk environment for HIV/AIDS than the outside world, whereas inmates perceive the opposite to be true. For prison staff, the main distinction between work and nonwork environments is that work brings staff into contact with inmates. Staff may perceive inmates as more likely to be HIV-seropositive than individuals contacted outside of prison; because of the widespread belief that HIV/AIDS risk behaviors are endemic in prisons, correctional staff may perceive a higher self-risk of HIV/AIDS (McKee et al., 1995). For both staff and inmates, greater concern about and perceived risk of HIV/AIDS were associated with a lower tolerance for interacting with people with HIV/AIDS and more support for strict social control measures against people with HIV/AIDS.

Mahaffey and Marcus (1995) examined correctional officers' views and attitudes about working with inmates with AIDS. Their purpose was to find out whether knowledge, worry, homophobia, and general attitudes toward people with AIDS were related to the correctional officers' specific attitudes toward working with inmates who were HIV-positive. One hundred fifty-three officers at three prisons in Texas were administered the AIDS in Prison Scale, the AIDS Attitude Scale, an HIV/AIDS knowledge test, and a homophobia scale. Correctional officers who had more positive attitudes about people with AIDS, who were more knowledgeable about HIV/AIDS, and who were older were more likely to have more positive views about working with inmates with HIV/AIDS. Most of the officers expressed at least some concerns about working with inmates with AIDS. Education programs that address negative attitudes about persons with AIDS may help improve the conditions of HIV-infected inmates.

Allard et al. (1992) conducted a self-administered questionnaire survey with the staff of half-way houses, probation agencies, and prison staff to determine the level of factual knowledge and personal attitudes of the staff of correctional facilities towards HIV and related infections. Knowledge was measured through the percentage of correct answers obtained. Attitudes were categorized as "fear of working with possibly infected persons," "desire to identify and isolate infected persons," and "acceptance of same-gender sexual behavior." The categories were measured with a Likert-type scale. Results suggest that most participants had good general knowledge of terminology (87.9 percent) and accurate concepts about infections (94.9 percent).

However, accurate knowledge of modes of transmission and preventive measures in the workplace was 58.9 percent. Prison officers and older correctional facility staff had the lowest scores on these questions ($p \sim .05$), while prison officers alone had the most negative attitudes ($p \sim .0001$). Generally better knowledge of modes of transmission and preventive measures was a predictor of positive attitudes ($p \sim .0001$). Allard et al. (1992) concluded that correctional staff enrolled in the AIDS education programs had good general knowledge of HIV and infections but lacked critical information on modes of transmission and preventive measures in the workplace. Since this latter type of knowledge is associated with more positive attitudes, it tends to support the hypothesis that education improves attitudes.

Gaughwin et al. (1990) conducted a systematic interview of 20 percent of the prison officers and an interview of 50 percent of the inmates in an Australian prison to evaluate the differences between the inmates and the prison staff in their knowledge and attitudes about HIV. They found that both inmates and prison officers think that information about AIDS has not resulted in substantial reduction in some risk behaviors, particularly injection drug use. A majority of inmates and prison officers think that inmates are indeed worried about getting HIV in prison, yet many inmates and staff think that those who engage in risk behaviors are not particularly worried.

HIV/AIDS Educational Programs in Prison Setting

The support of correctional officers and jail staff is crucial to the success of the educational programs. Officers can reduce the effectiveness of an HIV/AIDS education program. For example, they can sabotage inmate attendance at scheduled classes or release them slowly from cells or living areas so that hour-long sessions have only a few actual minutes with everyone in attendance. Staff can even stigmatize "inmates who attend or [staff can] loudly proclaim inaccurate 'facts' about HIV transmission, without accepting even diplomatic corrections from inmates recently educated" (Baxter, 1991, p. 49).

A possible policy for correctional institutions is the improvement of education for correctional staff. Education about AIDS has been a primary preventive response to the HIV-1 epidemic. The educational programs in correctional institutions are intended to reduce transmission of HIV by influencing the knowledge, attitudes, and behaviors of persons at high risk for the disease. A strategy for averting obstacles that relate to correctional staff is to provide a comprehensive orientation session that includes basic AIDS education and an overview of the program for inmates. In addition to giving useful and accurate information about HIV transmission and AIDS, this strategy acknowledges that the staff can strengthen the impact of the inmates' education program by being informed and supportive of behavior changes themselves.

Many correctional systems have implemented programs of AIDS education (Zimmerman et al., 1991). For example, 98 percent responding to the NIJ survey of correctional facilities reported that they provided AIDS education to correctional staff (Mahaffey & Marcus, 1995). However, these statistics may be misleading since prisons provided mandatory AIDS education to staff during orientation, and only half of these systems required updates in AIDS education. Previous NIJ reports also have questioned the quantity and quality of AIDS education in correctional facilities (Mahaffey & Marcus, 1995). Furthermore, evaluations of AIDS education programs and assessments of knowledge about AIDS among prison officers are sparse. Until recently, there were no published studies investigating the nature of effectiveness of the training provided to the staff of correctional facilities.

Although AIDS educational programs for correctional officers in prisons are virtually universal, there is still considerable misinformation and illogical fear about HIV/AIDS among correctional staffs. The most striking example of this misinformation may be correctional officers who fear casual transmission of the AIDS virus, even though AIDS cannot be casually transmitted. Research with health care workers has indicated minimal risk in exposure to human bodily fluid; yet according to NIJ reports, the fear of exposure to HIV through bodily fluids is a primary concern of correctional officers. Although there have been no job-related cases of HIV infection among American or Canadian correctional officers, fear of casual transmission persists; overall, concerns about HIV infection have not declined in recent years. Providing factual information about the transmission of HIV may be necessary, but not sufficient, to eliminate illogical fears (Mahaffey & Marcus, 1995).

Basic Approach

Corrections officials are likely to interact with HIV-infected individuals during work activities. They retain authority for deciding which procedures to implement to reduce the risk factors. Since only scant data exist on risk perception and behavior change among inmates, this survey provides new insights in this area. Also, syphilis, gonorrhea, and chlamydia are found to be potential risk factors for HIV disease (Cohen, Scribner, Clark, & Cory, 1992); thus STDs and HIV/AIDS factors should be considered together. Therefore, the results from the system interviews to be discussed in this chapter have important policy-related implications, especially in evaluating the current HIV/AIDS risk-reduction programs in the four correctional institutions surveyed.

The basic methodological approach involved identifying a sample of correctional staff (see Table 7.1) from each of the four institutions and soliciting their involvement as interviewees for this exploratory inquiry. An effort was made to secure a mix of personnel classifications, although the majority of the respondents were correctional officers. A research team member was trained by staff from the Centers for Disease Control and Prevention to implement the interview schedule. This training took place over three days and included both didactic and supervised hands-on interviewing experience. An instrument (Systems Interview Protocol) was designed after several interactions with the health provider personnel at the correctional facilities. The instrument sought to capture information from correctional staff relative to their perceptions about HIV/AIDS issues in the prison setting. Most of the questions were open-ended and designed to have the respondents free associate in terms of their views.

The semistructured interviews typically spanned a 45–75 minute period in a comfortable location within the facilities. The selection of the respondents was less random than that for the inmates reported in Chapter Six; thus it should be considered a convenience sample. The completed interviews were shipped to the university-based investigators in Atlanta, Georgia, where data coding, entry, and analysis took place. The reported results were formatted for simple frequencies.

Table 7.1. Occupational Classification of Respondents (*n* = 65).

Types of Occupations	n	percent
Administrator assistant	5	7.7 %
Nursing staff	8	12.3
Correctional staff	28	43.1
Social worker/psychologist	7	10.7
Teacher	2	3.1
Health educator	10	15.4
Administrator	5	7.7

Source: Braithwaite & Mayberry, 1996.

Survey Results

The System Interview Protocol surveys the staff ($n = 65$) attitudes toward HIV/AIDS risk-reduction programs in four correctional institutions: a West Coast juvenile detention facility (27.7 percent of the respondents), a West Coast male prison (24.6 percent), a rural southern boot camp (23.1 percent), and a Midwestern county jail (24.6 percent). The majority of the respondents were female personnel (66.2 percent). More than half of the interviewees were African American (56.3 percent), with 25 percent whites, 12.5 percent Hispanic, 1.6 percent Asian, and 4.7 percent others. About half of the interviewees were between age twenty-five and forty. The sample included people from a variety of jobs at the institutions, but 26.2 percent were correctional officers, which is the plurality in this sample. Fifty-seven percent of the staff surveyed had been in their current positions (at the time of interview) for less than three years. Fifty-one percent had never contacted any incarcerated populations before they came to their current working institutions.

Knowledge of Client Population

This section of the questionnaire probed staff knowledge and opinions of the incarcerated population. Most of the staff ($n = 62$, 95.4 percent) answered yes to whether there are different subgroups in the prison population. When asked which group of respondents ($n = 65$) they felt most knowledgeable and comfortable talking about, they did not indicate any distinct difference in their preferences by gender or age groups.

Staff Perceptions of Inmates' Risk for HIV/STDs

This section analyzes staff perceptions of risk for HIV infection and sexually transmitted diseases among the incarcerated. Of the sixty-four interviewees who were asked if the specific group (served at their respective prisons) were at risk for HIV infection before coming into the current correctional institution, fifty-nine (92.2 percent) respondents said yes. An even higher percentage (96.9 percent) of the staff responded similarly when considering prior risk for STDs. The behaviors that place the incarcerated group at risk for HIV infection were perceived by staff to include unsafe sex, drugs/alcohol, attitude, tattooing, and lack of knowledge. Staff's perception of the behavior that is most responsible for STDs is unsafe sex (63.5 percent of the respondents), followed by drugs/alcohol, lack of knowledge, prostitution, and tattooing (see Table 7.2).

According to staff perceptions, the leading factor contributing to HIV risk-taking behaviors is drugs/alcohol (26.7 percent), followed by lack of knowledge (16.7 percent), unsafe sex (13.3 percent), environmental conditions (11.7 percent), educational level (1.7 percent), prostitution (1.7 percent), and others (25 percent). Factors contributing to STDs risk-taking behaviors are drugs/alcohol (19.0 percent), unsafe sex (15.5 percent), lack of knowledge (15.5 percent), environmental (13.8 percent), economic reasons (3.4 percent), educational level (1.7 percent), prostitution (1.7 percent). See Table 7.3.

Education was identified as the most relevant tool (47.5 percent) that would help the inmate population reduce their risk for

Table 7.2. Behaviors Placing Inmates at Risk for HIV Infection and STDs.

Factors	HIV (n = 51)		STDs (n = 52)	
	n	%	n	%
Unsafe sex	31	60.8 %	33	63.5 %
Drugs/alcohol	12	23.5	9	17.3
Lack of knowledge	1	2.0	1	1.9
Tattooing	1	2.0	1	1.9
Attitude	1	2.0	1	1.9
Prostitution	—	—	1	1.9
Other	5	9.8	6	11.5
Total	51	100	52	100

*Source:*Braithwaite & Mayberry, 1996.

Table 7.3. Factors Contributing to HIV and STDs Risk-Taking Behaviors.

Factors	HIV (n = 60)		STDs (n = 58)	
	n	%	n	%
Unsafe sex	8	13.3 %	9	15.5 %
Drugs/alcohol	16	26.7	11	19.0
Lack of knowledge	10	16.7	9	15.5
Educational level	2	3.3	1	1.7
Economic reasons	1	1.7	2	3.4
Environmental	7	11.7	8	13.8
Prostitution	1	1.7	1	1.7
Other	15	25.0	17	29.3
Total	60	100	58	100

Source: Braithwaite & Mayberry, 1996.

HIV infection. Condom distribution (23.7 percent) was second. Other suggestions include drug treatment (10.2 percent), abstinence/control (5.1 percent), and nothing (5.1 percent). Almost the same results were evident for STDs risk-taking behaviors (see Table 7.4).

Inmate Perceptions of Risk According to Staff

This section probes staff perceptions of the inmates' own perceptions about HIV and STD risks. According to the data, the majority (67.2 percent) of the staff think that inmates do not consider themselves at risk for HIV infection. But 62.5 percent of the staff think that inmates know that they are at risk of STDs. It is evident that the staff perceive that inmates are more aware of the risks for STDs than for HIV. Factors considered as helpful to reduce HIV risks are condoms (42.6 percent), job skills (13.1 percent), drug rehabilitation (8.2 percent), HIV education (3.3 percent), and a steady income (1.6 percent). Factors for reducing STD risks

Table 7.4. Tools for HIV/STDs Risk Reduction.

Factors	HIV		STDs	
	n	%	n	%
Education	28	47.5 %	30	51.7 %
Condom distribution	14	23.7	14	24.1
Abstinence/control	3	5.1	2	3.4
Drug treatment	6	10.2	5	8.6
Nothing	3	5.1	3	5.2
Other	5	8.5	4	6.9
Total	59	100	58	100

Source: Braithwaite & Mayberry, 1996.

included condoms (42.6 percent), HIV education (13.1 percent), drug rehabilitation (6.6 percent), school (1.6 percent), and contraceptives (1.6 percent); see Table 7.5. According to the staff, several factors are considered by the inmates as barriers for them to reduce the risks for HIV and STDs.

Staff Recommendations for Program Development

This section addresses staff opinions on how to construct a program to help reduce the risk behaviors for HIV and STDs. For HIV, sex education is the most frequent recommendation (73 percent). Other proposed methods include education about human sexuality at an early age, free contraceptives, and emphasis on values and self-control. It was felt that the most important intervention program should be education (65.1 percent), followed distantly by recommendations to use condoms (9.5 percent). As for STDs, 90.5 percent agreed that there should not be much difference in the approach for the prevention of STD infection.

Perceived factors that make it hard to implement an HIV/AIDS program within correctional institutions are unwillingness of inmates (23.1 percent), staff needs/constraints (18.5 percent), administrative problems (18.5 percent), financial problems

Table 7.5. Inmates' Risk-Reduction Strategies for HIV and STDs.

Factors	HIV (n = 61)		STDs (n = 61)	
	n	%	n	%
Condoms	26	42.6 %	26	42.6 %
Job skills	8	13.1	—	—
School	—	—	1	1.6
HIV education	2	3.3	8	13.1
Steady income	1	1.6	—	—
Contraceptives	—	—	1	1.6
Drug abuse cure	5	8.2	4	6.6
Other	19	31.1	21	34.4
Total	61	100	61	100

Source: Braithwaite & Mayberry, 1996.

(10.8 percent), and insufficient staff training (1.5 percent). According to the survey, the best methods for overcoming barriers to implementing HIV/AIDS programs are educating employees (24.2 percent), educating inmates (16.1 percent), increasing staff (9.7 percent), and increasing funding (4.8 percent).

Factors that make it easier to conduct HIV/AIDS programs in the institutions, according to staff, include facility environment (39.1 percent), familiarity with inmates (14.1 percent), and type of client environment (10.9 percent). That "inmates want the program" only accounts for a very small percentage (1.6 percent) in the opinion of the staff. Effective ways to make it easier to provide HIV/AIDS programs included to educate inmates (39 percent), produce education programs (16.9 percent), educate staff (8.5 percent), and educate both inmates and staff (3.4 percent).

Assessment of Current Program

This section reports on the assessment of current HIV/AIDS programs in prison facilities. The majority of the staff (about 71 percent) indicate that their institutions offer HIV/AIDS education to both staff and inmates. The survey shows that most of the programs (81.3 percent) are relatively new, in existence for fewer than five years. The question "Does the institution have a written policy regarding HIV/AIDS education programs?" had a very low response rate (49.2 percent); however, the majority of the respondents (71.9 percent) answered yes. Among the existing programs, 11.1 percent are mandatory, 5.6 percent are optional, and 2.8 percent are conducted as orientation, while a very high percentage (27.8 percent) are mandatory for staff. With regard to schedules, 72 percent agree that there is a standard HIV/AIDS education curriculum at their institutions. The objectives of these programs are quite different, according to the survey. For example, 40.5 percent state that the objective is to educate inmates, while 14.3 percent state it is to educate staff, and 7.1 percent to educate both inmates and staff. Some (11.9 percent) state it is to prevent risky behavior. Others (7.1 percent) even consider it as a universal precaution.

The survey shows that the content of the program seems to be the same for different inmate groups, since 81.2 percent of the staff think that there is no difference in the contents. As to the question of who conducts the education program, 37.5 percent of the staff think it is the health educators. Other agents are medical doctors and registered nurses (15 percent), staff (15 percent), inmates (15 percent), health/social services (12.5 percent), and staff and inmates (2.5 percent).

Analysis of the questionnaire revealed some inconsistencies in perception of method and location for program delivery (see Table 7.6). The majority (72.1 percent) agree that the education program is delivered in a group form. Only 11.6 percent admit that it is done in one-to-one form. Still, 11.6 percent think it is done in both group and one-to-one forms. As to the settings in which the programs are provided, 87.9 percent indicate the classroom, 2.4 percent in the auditorium, 2.4 percent in the exam room, and 7.3 percent in other settings. The most popular materials used in the programs are videos (82.5 percent), brochures and pamphlets (15 percent), and lectures (2.5 percent).

The staff were also asked to comment on available programs and services for inmates. In addition to the HIV/AIDS programs in the institutions, some other educational programs are sometimes available, such as general education diploma (GED, 45.1

Table 7.6. Method and Location for Program Delivery.

	How (n = 43)			Where (n = 41)	
	n	%		n	%
One-on-one	5	11.6 %	Classroom	36	87.9 %
Group	31	72.1	Auditorium	1	2.4
Both	5	11.6	Exam room	1	2.4
Other	2	4.7	Other	3	7.3
Total	43	100		41	100

Source: Braithwaite & Mayberry, 1996.

percent), basic education (15.7 percent), vocational training (2 percent), and others (37.3 percent). According to the survey, 75 percent reported that the correctional institutions provide general medical treatment for inmates, and 3.6 percent admitted there is dental care service available to inmates; but the percentage for psychiatric care is quite low (1.8 percent). Finally, 5.4 percent reported there were no medical services offered to inmates.

Discussion

This survey shows that some of the staff have accurate knowledge about HIV infection. Correctional staff generally perceived education as a main tool to reduce inmate risk for HIV/STDs. Chi-square tests indicate that respondents did not differ by gender, race, or age except on two occasions. One is concerned with staff-perceived factors that could reduce the inmates' risk for HIV. There was a statistically significant difference between male and female personnel ($x^2(5) = 13.623$, $p = .018$). The other factor that would make it hard for inmates to reduce their risks for HIV is evidenced by marginal differences across race groups ($x^2(42) = 19.757$, $p = .072$).

It is apparent that staff perceive their own need for education about HIV/AIDS as an important dimension of their work environment. Such training will facilitate a more wholesome environment between staff and inmates. Even though many of the staff had accurate knowledge about HIV/STDs infection, educational programs in prison should continue to be an integral component of new-employee orientation.

The survey results also confirm perceptions held by correctional personnel that factors contributing to HIV and STD risk-taking behaviors are activities not condoned by the institution. Same-gender sex, drugs, and alcohol account for a combined 74 percent of the perceived risk. While correctional personnel identify these areas as risk, they are able to dismiss these areas from active programming since the areas are not condoned by the institutional policy. Thus the staff underestimate such behavior and give little to no attention for appropriate intervention and/or prevention at the institutions.

Consistently, correctional staff indicate that there is a lack of appropriate knowledge among inmates that contributes to their high-risk status for HIV and STDs. Yet there was little emphasis given to the need to promote education and prevention activities for inmates among the staff survey respondents. This lack of health promotion among this group may be indicative of how they identify their primary mission within the correctional system: the security function, as opposed to a rehabilitation function, typically dominates. This is a universal observation across correctional settings. Since this is the case, the role of the rehabilitation, social-psychological, and health provider staff persons within these institutions is secondary, which makes the opportunities for advancing innovative prevention programs a lesser priority when contrasted with other institutional priorities (usually of a security nature).

It is difficult to interpret why correctional staff perceive inmates as being more knowledgeable about the risk of STDs (62.5 percent) and less knowledgeable about the risk of HIV (67.2 percent). Perhaps it is the fact that STDs have historically been recognized as a disease and HIV is a relatively new phenomenon (since 1985); it may be that a more global recognition of risk has been internalized in the correctional staff's perceptions. Other literature across institutionalized and noninstitutionalized populations suggests that most high-risk groups have the knowledge but find it extremely difficult to change behaviors to be consistent with what they know.

What is also less clear is why correctional staff advance the idea that sex education should receive emphasis for programmatic areas, while again ignoring the high transmission risk associated with needle-sharing behaviors. Moreover, correctional staff recognize that the use of condoms is another effective strategy for risk reduction among inmates; yet virtually none of the staff would even suggest a policy research effort on this subject for fear of reprisals.

The correctional staff also perceived the inmates and their prevention needs as being a unitary factor, with little credence given to culture or ethnicity as a factor for differential curriculum or program development. While it is true that much of the accurate information about HIV/AIDS prevention is appropriate for all groups, irrespective of race, gender, or ethnicity, there are many cultural considerations that must be acknowledged to have an effective prevention program. For example, the *machismo* that exists among many Hispanic youths precludes them from using condoms. This becomes a cultural factor that will require investigation by multidisciplinary scientists—anthropologists, psychologists, and sociologists—to find plausible, culturally relevant, and effective intervention approaches. For correctional administrations to be effective in aiding the effort to combat the HIV pandemic as a public health concern will require more creative and risk-taking policy initiatives.

Chapter Eight

Legal and Legislative Issues

Since the mid-1980s, there has been a significant amount of litigation and legislative activity related to HIV/AIDS in correctional facilities. Cases involve inmate challenges to correctional systems' policies and practices regarding HIV testing, housing, and correctional management of inmates with HIV, disclosure of HIV-related information, and medical and psychosocial services. The courts have also addressed the right of inmates to live free from assault and from the risk of contracting HIV through coercive sexual acts (Burris, 1992). There have also been criminal cases filed for alleged HIV transmission and sentencing decisions in which HIV status played a role or in which defendants asked that their HIV status be considered. Legislative activity has centered on mandatory HIV antibody testing of all inmates or in certain circumstances, as well as disclosure of inmates' HIV status to correctional authorities and offenders' victims.

Several general themes emerge from the case law. While segregation of asymptomatic HIV-infected inmates is on the decline, courts generally continue to uphold correctional systems' housing policies as well as prohibitions against food-service and other work assignments for those found to be HIV-positive or to have other infectious diseases. Legislation imposing mandatory HIV testing of all inmates has declined since the late 1980s, but there has been a recent proliferation of laws calling for mandatory testing of convicted (and, in some instances, accused) sex offenders as well as some laws providing for the disclosure of inmates' HIV status to correctional authorities.

Protection from HIV Infection Through Coercive or Assaultive Acts of Other Inmates

The possibility of a prisoner being infected with HIV through a rape or sexual assault is perhaps the most explosive legal and moral issue related to HIV/AIDS in correctional facilities. At this writing, there have been no cases in which an inmate was able to establish that he or she acquired HIV in prison due to a rape or sexual assault. However, a number of such allegations have been lodged. In such instances, prisoners can bring suit against the responsible officials or government entities under 42 U.S.C. § 1983 (Siegal, 1992).

Perhaps the most significant case to come before the courts in recent years with relevance to HIV/AIDS in prisons is *Farmer* v. *Brennan* (1994). The U.S. Supreme Court's ruling in *Farmer* v. *Brennan* may help to define the obligation of corrections officials to protect prisoners from injury at the hands of fellow prisoners. By extension, this holding could apply to cases of HIV transmission through rape or sexual assault. In June 1994, the high court ruled that prison officials may be found liable for failing to protect an inmate from violence at the hands of other prisoners if the officials did not act when they knew of a "substantial risk of physical harm." The Court's 9–0 ruling came in the case of a transsexual federal prisoner whose suit against prison officials had been dismissed by two lower federal courts in Indiana. The ruling gave the prisoner a chance to show at trial that the beatings and rapes he suffered were the result of prison officials' "deliberate indifference" to his need for special protection. "Deliberate indifference" is the governing standard for assertions that prison conditions represent cruel and unusual punishment under the Constitution (*Wilson* v. *Seiter*, 1991). The standard was first enunciated with regard to medical care in *Estelle* v. *Gamble* (1976).

The Farmer case (*Farmer* v. *Brennan*, 1994), which clearly established the duty of prison officials to protect inmates from fellow inmates as well as from officers, still requires a showing by the prisoner that the officials knew of the risk and failed to take reasonable measures to prevent injury to the prisoner. However, an inmate can prevail without proving that he or she had warned officials of a particular threat or that officials believed that harm was about to befall a particular inmate. Circumstantial evidence can suffice to demonstrate that officials had the requisite knowledge, and the judge or jury "may conclude that a prison official knew of a substantial risk from the very fact that the risk was obvious." Another important aspect of this decision is that it admits evidence of a correctional system's "subjective intent" to allow conditions to exist in which inmates might suffer harm or abuse at the hands of their fellows. The admissibility of such evidence allows plaintiffs' access to internal memoranda and other documents in which subjective intent may be documented.

Mandatory Testing

Mandatory HIV testing of prisoners may be in place pursuant to state law, executive order, or correctional system policy. In most cases, such as *Dunn* v. *White* (1989, 1990), courts have upheld mandatory testing of inmates on the ground that such policies are "reasonably related to legitimate penological interests," the principle for testing the constitutionality of correctional policies enunciated by the U.S. Supreme Court in *Turner* v. *Safley* (1987) (Belbot & del Carmen, 1991).

In *Walker* v. *Sumner* (1990), the Federal Appeals Court for the Ninth Circuit reversed a district court's summary judgment concerning Nevada's mandatory HIV testing policy, holding that the state had offered only conclusory allegations that its policy furthered a legitimate penological interest. However, upon rehearing in the district court, the court was satisfied that evidence of legitimate penological interest had been adduced by the state, and the testing policy was allowed to stand.

In *Ormond* v. *Mississippi* (1989), the Mississippi Supreme Court, basing its decision on *Dunn,* ruled that Mississippi did not violate the rights of an inmate when it treated him for gonorrhea. The court in *Dunn* affirmed the state's contention that its treatment of inmates outweighed their privacy interests, in light of its duty to prohibit the spread of sexually transmittable diseases in the prison. In *Dunn* v. *White* (1989/1990), noted the Mississippi Supreme Court, the appeals panel "balanced the scope of the particular intrusion, the manner in which it is conducted, the justification for initiating it, and the place in which it is conducted," and ultimately found "HIV testing permissible and not in violation of the Fourth Amendment or privacy interests." In declaring the related portion

of Ormond's appeal without merit, the court ruled that his gonorrhea treatment had been provided in the legitimate interest of
"protecting inmates at the jail from a communicable disease and
in treating and providing for the health of inmates. . . . The State's
interests outweigh the privacy interests of the defendant, and the
method chosen to administer the treatment for gonorrhea was a
proper mechanism" (*Ormond* v. *Mississippi,* 1989).

Testing in Response to Incidents

Case law generally affirms correctional systems' compulsory testing of inmates involved in assaults or other incidents posing risk
of HIV transmission. On the other hand, inmates seeking to be
tested after they were involved in potential transmission incidents
have not fared as well in the courts.

In *Lile* v. *Tippecanoe County Jail* (1992), a case brought *pro se*
(without assistance of counsel), a federal district court in Indiana
found that inmates' rights were not violated by a jail's failure to
provide inmates with HIV antibody tests after they were splattered
with the blood of a fellow inmate.

Connor v. *Foster* (1993) involved an arrestee who alleged that he
was involuntarily tested for HIV after his arrest, in part because one
of the arresting officers had been pricked during the arrest by a
hypodermic needle in the arrestee's pocket. The court ruled that
state law (*Illinois Compiled Statutes,* 1992) explicitly sanctioned the
testing of the arrestee. Effective January 1, 1990, Illinois amended
its statutes to dispense with the need for written informed consent
to conduct an HIV test "[w]hen a law enforcement officer is
involved in the line of duty in a direct skin or mucous membrane
contact with the blood or bodily fluids of an individual which is of
a nature that may transmit HIV as determined by a physician in his
medical judgment" (pp. 727, 730).

The court ruled that because the puncture that was suffered in
conducting the search clearly contained the potential for transmission of HIV, under Illinois law no written consent was needed
to force the arrestee to undergo an HIV antibody test.

Similarly, in *Johnetta* v. *Municipal Court* (1990), a California
appellate court upheld the state law requiring HIV antibody testing of persons alleged to have been involved in possible transmission incidents with peace officers or employees of custodial

facilities. In this case, brought by a defendant accused of biting a court officer, the court held that such a mandatory test did not constitute an unreasonable search and seizure. There is a possibility—albeit remote—that HIV can be transmitted through a bite, the court wrote, and therefore the assailant's test results "would be useful in treating the bitten officer and in easing the officer's anxiety."

In 1994, the Illinois Appellate Court for the Fourth District upheld a ruling of the Circuit Court of Livingston County ordering that a prisoner be tested for HIV despite opposition to the test by the Illinois Department of Corrections. "Jane Doe," a correctional officer at the Dwight Illinois Correctional Center, was bitten twice by an inmate. Doe had alleged that a first test of the inmate was inadequate and had asked the trial court to direct the Department of Corrections to conduct a second test. The court stated that while it is not its duty to supervise the day-to-day operations of prisons, this was not a case of directing what meals should be served or what hours should be kept. Instead, according to a concurring opinion, the case "involves providing proper information to a victim of a wrongdoing" ("Illinois Appeals Court . . . ," 1994).

Anderson v. *Murdaugh* (1992/1993), a federal district court case from South Carolina, considered the HIV antibody testing of those convicted of criminal sexual conduct. In *Anderson,* a *pro se* plaintiff who had been convicted of the kidnapping and rape of a convenience store operator contended that his Fourth Amendment rights were violated when he was forced to undergo a test ordered by a state circuit judge. Citing a similar decision in *State* v. *Farmer* (1991), the *Anderson* court held that this testing met the statutory requirement. The law provides for mandatory testing only of persons convicted of crimes involving sexual battery which exposed the victim to the convicted person's bodily fluids.

The case above concerned a person who had been convicted of a sex offense. Considerable controversy has arisen over statutes proposed or enacted in some jurisdictions that would compel testing of persons charged but not yet convicted of such offenses.

Confidentiality

The confidentiality of HIV antibody test results and other information on inmates' HIV status has also been the subject of litigation. In *Doe* v. *Meachum* (1989), a Connecticut case challenging the correctional system's management of HIV-infected inmates, a federal district court recognized the privacy interests of inmates in their medical records. Through the use of protective orders, the court limited disclosure of those records to individuals involved in the litigation who had need for access to them. The court also allowed HIV-positive inmates to testify under fictitious names.

In *Doe* v. *City of New York* (1994), the Federal Appeals Court for the Second Circuit reversed a district court opinion and held that "individuals who are infected with the HIV virus clearly possess a constitutional right to privacy regarding their condition." The *Doe* court wrote that this is a right to "confidentiality, rather than autonomy and independence in decision-making"; "The right to confidentiality includes the right to protection regarding information about the state of one's health." The plaintiff's entry into a conciliation agreement on his discrimination claim filed with the City Commission on Human Rights did not constitute a waiver of his privacy rights. While this case did not involve an inmate or correctional setting, it raises important issues regarding disclosure of HIV status. The confidentiality of HIV antibody test results has also been the subject of litigation within and outside of the prison context.

On the other hand, a federal appeals court ruled in *Doe* v. *Wigginton* (1994) that the disclosure to a correctional officer of the inmate's HIV status did not violate the inmate's right to privacy. In its decision, the court relied on a 1981 Sixth Circuit case holding that the disclosure of juveniles' "social histories" does not violate the right of privacy and that the Constitution "does not encompass a general right to nondisclosure of private information."

Capaldini v. *Sheriff of San Francisco County* (1991) was a California case that considered the constitutionality of the San Francisco County Sheriff's Department's plan to comply with California Proposition 96. Proposition 96 was a voter-approved 1988 law that required medical workers in jails and prisons to disclose the names of inmates with communicable diseases to correctional workers responsible for supervising them. After a lengthy pretrial exchange of discoverable material in the case, plaintiff's counsel concluded that, with some modifications, the county sheriff's implementation plan, which placed tight controls on distribution of the information, was acceptable. Counsel for the plaintiff entered into a stipulation with the sheriff's department, and the case was dismissed without prejudice to the plaintiffs (Matthew Coles, staff attorney, ACLU Foundation of Northern California, personal communication, 1993).

Segregation and Housing Assignments

As discussed earlier, the trend in corrections is to mainstream HIV-positive prisoners—that is, to house them in the general prison population. Nonetheless, lawsuits concerning segregation of HIV-positive inmates continue to be quite common, with the courts generally, but not universally, issuing rulings upholding correctional policies whether or not these are in line with the trend away from segregation.

A number of court decisions have upheld correctional systems' policies to mainstream HIV-infected inmates. One of the first major cases was *Glick* v. *Henderson* (1988), in which a prisoner contended that prison administrators' failure to segregate inmates infected with HIV from the general prisoner population constituted a failure to protect the health and safety of noninfected inmates. The *Glick* court held that the complaint did not state a claim of "deliberate indifference," the constitutional standard, because the plaintiff did not show a pervasive risk of contracting HIV, and that his claims were based on "unsubstantiated fears and ignorance." This reasoning, and deference to correctional officials' decisions regarding the best housing policies for their systems, have been followed in numerous subsequent cases.

Myers v. *Maryland Division of Correction* (1992) involved a demand by Maryland inmates for mandatory segregation of HIV-positive inmates. In a ruling denying plaintiffs' claims under the cruel-and-unusual-punishment clause of the Eighth Amendment, the district court held that the Division of Correction's programs and policies, including those adopted since the lawsuit was instituted, did not violate their plaintiffs' rights. The court acknowledged that a risk of HIV infection existed under the current policies, but it held that the plaintiffs had failed to present evidence that defendants had been deliberately indifferent to that risk in formulating their policies. To the contrary, the court ruled, it is undisputed that the policies and programs instituted by the Maryland correctional system fall well within the norm of those instituted by other state prison systems. They also conform to applicable community standards outside the prison context.

In *Muhammad* v. *Federal Bureau of Prisons* (1991/1992), a U.S. district judge in Washington, D.C., rejected a federal inmate's request for a writ of mandamus compelling the Federal Bureau of Prisons to remove immediately all HIV-infected inmates from the general prison population. In dismissing the complaint, the judge stated that "[t]he remedy sought by plaintiff, that is, segregation of all inmates who test positive for HIV or have AIDS, is not a remedy available to the general public, and has not been found generally available to inmates in the courts" (District of Columbia Court, 1992, p. 8244).

The court noted that the Federal Bureau of Prisons maintains a policy under which HIV-positive inmates may be segregated "when there is reliable evidence that the inmate may engage in conduct posing a health risk to another person . . . " and that the approach is "consistent with the general medical understanding that AIDS is not spread through casual contact."

In *Johnson* v. *United States* (1993), a federal district court in Alabama ruled that placing the plaintiff in a cell with an HIV-infected inmate did not violate the Eighth Amendment prohibition against cruel and unusual punishment. The plaintiff alleged that his former cellmate tampered with his toothbrush, toothpaste, and razor blades. In addition, the plaintiff claimed that on several occasions he observed his cellmate's blood on their sink, toilet, and towels. Although the plaintiff did not allege that he contracted HIV from sharing facilities with his HIV-infected cellmate, he fears he may have contracted HIV from him. Additionally, Johnson complained that he was subjected to witnessing his cellmate's deteriorating condition and that during the two days prior to his cellmate's death, he was forced to feed and "sanitize" him. At the time of the court's decision, the plaintiff had tested negative for HIV three times since the cellmate's death.

In its decision, the *Johnson* court wrote that "to establish an Eighth Amendment claim, the evidence must show that the measure taken inflicted unnecessary and wanton pain and suffering . . . or was totally without penological justification" and that prison officials were deliberately indifferent to a condition of confinement which constitutes cruel and unusual punishment.

The court cited the declaration of Dr. Kenneth Moritsugu, the medical director of the Federal Bureau of Prisons:

The Bureau of Prisons does not segregate HIV-positive inmates. HIV-positive inmates remain in an institution's general population as long as they do not require hospitalization. The Bureau's emphasis on education, universal precautions, and professional management of HIV-positive inmates has rendered isolation unnecessary. . . . Inmates who are HIV-positive and who are believed to put other inmates or employees at risk (e.g., those who display intentional behavior that can result in the spread of the virus) are administratively separated from those whom they place at risk.

All Bureau of Prison inmates are informed of ways to avoid contracting AIDS. . . . Policy and training stress that individuals must respond to the presence of blood, semen, vaginal fluids, or any body fluids containing visible blood under the presumption that these fluids are contaminated. Inmates are informed that casual contact will not result in exposure to the virus. . . .

An inmate can have an HIV-positive roommate and not be at any risk of contracting the virus unless the inmates engage in high-risk behavior . . . [*Wilson v. Seiter,* 1991, p. 2321, 2324].

The *Johnson* (1993) court reasoned that as the prison rules prohibit the types of behavior that may result in transmission of HIV, those prisoners who follow the rules are not in significant danger of being infected. Therefore, prison officials' policy decisions not to segregate the HIV-infected inmates cannot be said to constitute deliberate indifference. The plaintiff had not been deprived of any basic need by the prison officials' actions. The plaintiff neither alleged that his former cellmate had engaged in high-risk conduct which would expose him to HIV, nor did the plaintiff allege any facts or allegations from which it might be inferred that the decision to house an HIV-infected inmate with the plaintiff evidenced a deliberate indifference to his serious medical needs or a culpable state of mind on the part of the defendants.

Courts have also upheld correctional systems' policies of segregating HIV infected inmates. For example, in *Harris v. Thigpen* (1991), the U.S. Circuit Court of Appeals for the Eleventh Circuit upheld the Alabama Department of Corrections' regulations requiring the HIV antibody testing of inmates and the segregation of those found to be HIV-positive. The Eleventh Circuit's decision held that the district court was correct in finding that the Alabama prison system was not deliberately indifferent to the medical and psychiatric needs of seropositive inmates. The appeals court also affirmed the district court's ruling that HIV-positive inmates' constitutionally protected privacy rights were not violated by Alabama prison policy requiring mandatory HIV testing and segregation. "Mandatory testing and segregation still apparently lie within the perimeter of an important correctional policy debate," wrote the appeals court. As such, it represents precisely the type of urgent problem of prison reform and prison administration with which the court is "ill equipped to deal," added the court.

The appeals court ruled that even if Alabama is in the minority, its combined policy of testing and segregating is connected to the legitimate goal of reducing HIV infection and reducing violence among inmates. Wrote the court, "It is inescapable that corrections systems should attempt to (1) prevent high risk behavior among inmates, (2) make reasonable efforts to protect all inmates from victimization, and (3) avoid any practices which could lead to unprotected blood exposure. The bounds of these duties as they relate to AIDS, and whether negligence or constitutional wrongs are involved, have not yet been clearly defined. At this early stage of the diagnosis and treatment of AIDS, these matters should be left in the hands of prison officials with the help of their medical staffs."

However, the appeals court in *Harris* v. *Thigpen* remanded to the district court the question of whether HIV-infected inmates should be entitled, under Section 504 of the Rehabilitation Act of 1973, to participate in more prison activities. Under the statute, courts have held that persons who are HIV infected are handicapped persons and entitled to "reasonable accommodation" of their needs in employment and other areas if they are "otherwise" qualified to participate in such activities or hold such positions. In remanding to the district court the issue of "whether the blanket exclusion of HIV-positive inmates from general prison population housing, educational, employment, community placement, and other programs violates Section 504 of the Rehabilitation Act," the Eleventh Circuit held that the district court had erred in failing to determine the risk of transmission not merely with regard to prison in general, but with regard to each program from which the appellants had been automatically excluded. The district court, the appeals court held, is obligated to determine whether reasonable accommodations by the Alabama Department of Corrections "could minimize such risk to an acceptable level" relying not on "general findings" but on a "particularized inquiry" with full findings of fact and conclusions of law as to each program and activity from which HIV-positive inmates are being excluded and a proper weighing of the dangers of transmission in each context.

The appeals court also directed the district court to reconsider whether lack of adequate access to the prison library denies HIV-infected inmates the right of access to courts, thus violating the First and Fourteenth Amendments. The parties continue to dispute the scope of the issues remanded to the district court, and as of this writing the case is not expected to come to trial for some time.

Derby v. *Allison* (1993/1996), a federal district court case from Iowa, involved an HIV-infected inmate's allegation that Iowa prison officials violated his constitutional rights to privacy, equal protection, free exercise of religion, and access to the courts when they ordered him medically segregated from the general population. In accordance with the communicable disease policy of the Iowa Department of Corrections, Derby was not initially segregated from the general population. Under the policy, inmates with communicable diseases such as AIDS are housed in general population unless they act in such a way as to heighten the risk of transmission to other inmates. In December 1992, Derby received a disciplinary report for having sexual contact with another inmate and for soliciting sex from others. Based upon a determination that Derby had engaged in sex with another inmate and the fact that he had two infectious diseases, AIDS and hepatitis, Derby was transferred to the Iowa State Penitentiary for the remainder of his term and placed in medical segregation there. Derby alleged that guards violated his constitutional right to privacy by telling fellow inmates that he had AIDS. He further alleged that a red medical segregation tag and infectious disease protocol posted on his cell violated his right to privacy and led inmates to threaten him out of fear of his illness.

A federal magistrate submitted a report and recommendation to the district court that was generally supportive of the actions of prison officials. The report recommended the following findings:

- Defendants did not violate Derby's rights by transferring him because an inmate has no constitutional right to a particular prison classification or status.
- Derby's medical segregation was not a pretext for punitive segregation and Derby received sufficient due process.
- Since the Supreme Court has held that inmates do not have an absolute right to participate in rehabilitation programs (*Moody* v. *Daggett*, 1976) Derby's rights were not violated by his transfer out of a facility with an alcohol and drug treatment program.
- There is no merit to Derby's equal protection claim that he was segregated because he is homosexual and afflicted with AIDS. On the contrary, Derby was segregated because his conduct posed a risk because of HIV transmission through solicited sexual contact. Thus, Derby was not "similarly situated" (the Constitutional test for an equal protection claim) to the general inmate population who do not engage in such risky conduct.
- Derby has not proven that unnamed guards told inmates about his AIDS status.

In January 1996, the district court upheld the magistrate's report and recommendations and dismissed Derby's case with prejudice.

A notable exception to courts' tendencies to uphold correctional systems' housing policies for HIV-infected inmates is *Nolley* v. *County of Erie* (1991), which represents an important decision against segregation. It involved an action by a former inmate infected with HIV against a correctional facility and various facility administrators, alleging constitutional and statutory violations in connection with her housing and other treatment. During three separate periods of incarceration, Nolley was placed in a segregated unit for mentally disturbed and suicidal inmates and denied access to the law library and religious services. She never developed AIDS; the decision to segregate Nolley was admittedly based solely on her HIV-positive status. Her housing assignment was never reviewed, and she was never afforded a hearing on it. The district court found that her segregation effectively disclosed her medical condition, violating her constitutional right to privacy, and lacked a legitimate penological purpose as defined in *Turner* v. *Safley* (1987). It reasoned that segregation is so remotely connected to the asserted goal of protecting general population inmates as to render the policy irrational and arbitrary.

Access to Programs

Issues regarding access of HIV-infected inmates to programs and work assignments have arisen under the Federal Rehabilitation Act of 1973 and the Americans with Disabilities Act (Gostin, 1992). Although a significant risk of transmission of HIV could justify exclusion of infected persons from jobs for which they are otherwise qualified (*School Board of Nassau County* v. *Arline,* 1987) the Ninth Circuit has found, based on reasonable medical judgment, that there is no significant risk of transmitting HIV disease except through "(1) intimate sexual contact with an infected person; (2) invasive exposure to contaminated blood or certain other bodily fluids; or (3) perinatal exposure (i.e., from mother to infant)" (*Chalk* v. *U.S. District Court,* 1988).

Despite these rulings, however, courts have generally upheld correctional systems' exclusion of HIV-infected inmates from various programs and assignments. In *Farmer* v. *Moritsugu* (1990), a federal district court in Wisconsin upheld the policy of the Federal Bureau of Prisons that prohibits HIV-infected inmates from working in prison hospitals or food services as a necessary measure to maintain order and security. The judge dismissed the inmates' complaint, ruling that there was no equal protection violation.

In *Gates* v. *Rowland* (1994), the Ninth Circuit Court of Appeals ruled that a district court had improperly ordered prison officials to allow HIV-positive inmates to work in prison food service. The ruling came in a case that considered a class-action lawsuit by prison inmates challenging conditions of confinement and segregation of HIV-infected inmates at the California Medical Facility at Vacaville. A subclass of HIV-positive inmates alleged that their segregation and exclusion from programs and work assignments violated the Federal Rehabilitation Act. A mediator brought in to resolve differences that had arisen regarding a consent decree in the original district court case recommended that the court prohibit the correctional system from excluding HIV-infected inmates from food-service jobs, absent a written determination that an individual inmate was not otherwise qualified to perform the job and that the defendant could not reasonably accommodate the inmate so that he would be able to perform the essential function of the job. The district court adopted these findings and held that the policy of excluding HIV-positive inmates from food service violated the Rehabilitation Act.

In *Gates* (1994), the issue before the appeals court was how the Rehabilitation Act was to be applied in a prison setting. Maintaining that there is no reason to believe Congress intended the Rehabilitation Act to apply to prison facilities without regard to the reasonable requirements of effective prison administration, the circuit court of appeals deemed the applicable standard for the review of statutory rights in a prison setting to be equivalent to the review of constitutional rights in the same setting, namely the standard of legitimate penological interest, set forth in *Turner* v. *Safley* (1987).

In reversing the district court, the Ninth Circuit stressed the particular sensitivity of prisoners to food service, which had often been the source of violence or riots. The court noted:

> The prisoners have no choice of where to eat. The prison authorities testified that if HIV seropositive inmates are placed in food service jobs, the other inmates will perceive a threat regardless of scientific research or medical pronouncements. When the transmission is by bodily fluids, such perceptions are particularly likely. Inmates fear that other inmates may do things to food that might be objectionable. If HIV seropositive inmates are placed in food service jobs, other inmates will think the worst . . . , that they will bleed into the food, spit into the food, or even worse. If the inmate population perceives a risk from the food they must eat, they will want the infected inmates removed from the food service jobs. If they have no assurance that the infected inmates are removed,

there may be violent actions against the inmates with the virus, inmates they perceive to have the virus, or the staff that permits the perceived risk [*Gates* v. *Rowland*, 1994, pp. 13523, 13542].

In response to the plaintiffs' contention that proper education concerning HIV transmission would remove the perceived risk, the court noted that many inmates are not motivated by rational thought and have irrational suspicions or phobias that education would not modify. In light of these findings, the appeals court ruled that Vacaville prison officials had provided a reasonable basis for the exclusion of HIV-positive inmates from food-service positions.

Adequacy of Medical Care for Inmates with HIV Disease

Much litigation focuses on the adequacy of medical care and associated services for inmates with HIV disease. Lawsuits have resulted in dramatic improvements in care in some prison systems. In Connecticut, for example, under a consent decree, Yale University Medical School has become heavily involved in HIV care in the prisons and the quality of care has improved dramatically as a result (*Doe* v. *Meachum*, 1989).

Elsewhere, it has been argued that medical care for inmates with HIV suffers from application of a double standard. In testimony before the National Commission on AIDS, Scott Burris of the Pennsylvania ACLU (American Civil Liberties Union) contrasted court findings in *Harris* v. *Thigpen* (1990) and other prison cases to that of *Weaver* v. *Reagan* (1988/1989), the leading case regarding the availability of zidovudine to Medicaid patients. In *Harris*, as in most other prison cases, the court held that inmates are not entitled to state-of-the-art medical care and that reasonable care according to community standards meets the constitutional requirement. By contrast, Burris notes that in *Weaver*, neither the trial court nor the court of appeals was deterred by medical disagreement about the utility of zidovudine and held that the drug must be provided under Medicaid coverage.

Inmates of New York with Human Immunodeficiency Virus v. *Cuomo* (1990) is a large federal class-action lawsuit, the outcome of which may have a profound impact on conditions of confinement for inmates with HIV disease in New York State. The plaintiffs are represented by four attorneys assisted by a number of medical experts on HIV. Plaintiffs are in the process of receiving the medical records of more than two hundred inmates and computer records for health care on the class. Attorneys are in direct contact with more than seven hundred HIV-positive inmates in the system and have received more than seventeen thousand AIDS surveillance forms (including multiple forms for some individuals). Early in the case the court refused to allow access to inmates' medical records without specific patient releases. Plaintiffs' counsel began deposing care providers during the spring of 1993, but at this writing trial is still probably several years away.

Cases Involving HIV Transmission

Criminal Charges

Despite the absence of any evidence that HIV has been transmitted through saliva, over the last several years at least four HIV-infected inmates have been prosecuted and convicted of attempted murder for biting or spitting on a correctional officer.

New Jersey inmate Gregory Dean Smith was serving a five-year term for robbery when he was sentenced to an additional twenty-five years in prison for biting a correctional officer. In 1993 the New Jersey Superior Court's Appellate Division upheld Smith's attempted murder conviction and sentence (*New Jersey* v. *Smith*, 1993). According to trial testimony, the incident occurred when Smith, after falling in his cell, was taken to a local hospital for an examination; he was accompanied by two corrections officers, who donned rubber gloves on being told the inmate was HIV-positive. The defendant reportedly became angry when hospital staff refused to take an X-ray of his back, and when the guards sought to get him into a patrol car for the return trip to jail, a scuffle ensued during which the guards' gloves came off. After biting one of the officers on the hand, Smith was reported to have said, "Now die, you pig! Die from what I have!"

In oral argument of the appeal, attorneys for the inmate had asserted that the guilty verdict and twenty-five-year prison sentence resulted from public hysteria regarding AIDS and would not have been applied to Smith were he not carrying HIV. By contrast, the prosecution maintained that whether HIV could be transmitted through a bite was legally irrelevant; it was the defendant's intent that mattered. Smith's attorneys argued that he "was as likely to have caused the death of . . . [corrections officers] by biting them as he was to have caused their deaths by sticking pins in dolls bearing their licenses" and that the court "has the solemn obligation of declaring that in the 1990's . . . no reasonable or ordinary person could possibly believe that the HIV virus can be transmitted by biting." Smith's attorneys also argued that "[a] threat by a person with AIDS to kill another by biting should convey precisely the same fear of death to an ordinary person as would a threat to kill by fly swatter, feather pillow, or incantation."

In its decision, the appellate court agreed with the prosecutor's contention that it did not matter whether HIV can actually be transmitted by biting as long as the inmate believed that it could. Its ruling included part of the jury instruction given by the trial court judge: "Impossibility is not a defense to the charge of attempted murder. That is because our law, our criminal statutes, punish conduct based on state of mind."

Texas inmate Curtis Weeks, serving a two-year sentence for robbery, received a sentence of ninety-nine years or life for spitting in an officer's face. A federal district court judge in Texas refused to overturn the life sentence. In her order in *Weeks v. Collins* (1994), the federal judge applied the Supreme Court standard that a court "must determine whether, after reviewing the evidence in the light most favorable to the prosecution, any rational trier of fact could have found the essential elements of the crime beyond a reasonable doubt." That evidence, the judge noted, included testimony that the inmate had HIV, that some people infected with HIV have the virus in their saliva, that blood might be in saliva because the inmate needed dental work and had just eaten, that the virus is transmitted through the mucous membrane, and that the inmate's saliva got inside the guard's nose, a mucous membrane. In *Weeks v. Collins*, attorneys for the inmate had urged the district court to recommend immediate dismissal of his "illegal, unconstitutional conviction and sentence," saying the state had "failed to prove an essential element of the crime of attempted murder." The pleading came in response to the state's motion for summary judgment in *Weeks* v. *Morales* (1993), a case considering a writ of habeus corpus filed by Weeks. In their brief to the court, attorneys for Weeks argued that the state failed to prove an essential element of the crime of attempted murder because there was no evidence establishing that spitting by an HIV-infected person can cause death. Attorneys for Weeks further argued that the state failed to demonstrate that Weeks acted with the capacity to commit the offense because it failed to offer any proof that Weeks' saliva contained HIV. While some legal scholars believed Weeks had a good argument, he made essentially the same one before a state appeals court, which rejected it in *Weeks* v. *State of Texas* (1992). In her ruling in *Weeks* v. *Collins* (1994), the district court judge also rejected the inmate's attorneys' request to take judicial notice of an advisory published in the *Texas Register* suggesting that biting and being bitten are not considered exposure to HIV unless blood is present. In 1995, the U.S. Circuit Court of Appeals for the Fifth Circuit affirmed the decision denying Weeks' petition for habeus corpus and upheld his conviction for attempted murder (*Weeks* v. *Scott,* 1995).

Civil Cases

In *Doe* v. *State of New York* (1992), the claimants, husband and wife, alleged that because corrections officers failed to restrain a hospital inmate, Mrs. Doe, a nurse, was pricked with a hypodermic needle and contracted HIV infection. In a ruling for the claimants, the husband and wife were awarded $4.3 million in damages, the husband was given an additional $1 million, and the judge indicated that after her death, the victim's survivors might bring a wrongful death suit for pecuniary injuries resulting from her death.

Indictment and Sentencing of Persons with HIV Disease

Whether and how the judicial system should consider HIV infection in its processing of persons accused and/or convicted of crimes remains a challenging question for the nation's criminal and appellate courts. Conflicting rulings appear largely related to the nature of the crime committed and to the nature of the defendant's illness. For example, while in recent years several courts have considered not prosecuting, or commuting the sentences of, defendants with HIV or AIDS who have been charged with or convicted of nonviolent crimes, other crimes such as having unprotected sex with teenagers are treated quite severely. In one such nonviolent offender case, *New York* v. *Larson* (1993), a majority of the Appellate Division of the New York Supreme Court, First Department, affirmed a lower court's dismissal of indictments against a man indicted for drug dealing. In its decision, the appellate division noted that at the time the trial court announced the dismissal, "the defendant's physical condition had progressively deteriorated during the pendency of the prosecution to the point that the defendant had become as thin as a rail and could hardly stand." The appellate division stated that the alleged criminality had been motivated by the suspect's need to feed his addiction and since that addiction was now being addressed in treatment, there was little risk of recidivism and no danger posed to the community.

In *Arizona* v. *John Wayne Ellevan* (1993), an Arizona appeals court ordered the resentencing of a convicted thief who is HIV-positive because his sixteen-year sentence amounted to life in prison. In its decision, the court noted that "[p]ositive HIV status is material to informed plea bargaining and sentence because it can transform into a life sentence a term of years that would otherwise end well within the recipient's probable life span." The inmate, John W. Ellevan, sought a resentencing on his conviction after learning while in prison that he was HIV-positive. A trial court judge had dismissed the inmate's petition saying that the inmate had failed to prove that he became infected before he was sentenced.

Rejecting the trial court's reasoning in a unanimous decision, the Arizona Court of Appeals held that the trial court had abused its discretion in failing to grant a resentencing. "Of two possible alternatives," wrote the court, "that petitioner was infected with HIV before or after sentencing the evidence introduced at the hearing tended only to support the first." The appeals court also noted that the state had offered no evidence to support its assertion that the prisoner could have become infected inside prison. The appeals court decision ordered the trial judge to resentence the prisoner in light of the discovery of his HIV-positive status.

In contrast, many courts are quite harsh in dealing with HIV-positive individuals who engage in unprotected sex. For example, in *Virginia* v. *Webb* (1994) a Petersburg, Virginia, court sentenced a twenty-eight-year-old HIV-positive man to ten years in prison for knowingly having unprotected sex with three teenage girls. Two of the girls had been infected with HIV, and one of the two was pregnant. Although Virginia has no legal precedent for the charges against Webb, the state looked to legal theories from other states where such persons have been convicted of attempted murder or assault with a deadly weapon. According to the charging attorney, Webb had known since 1988 that he was HIV-positive and "knew the importance of protected sex and disclosure to his sexual partners." In spite of this knowledge, the defendant continued to have unprotected sex with multiple partners without disclosing that he was HIV-positive.

Proving intent was a concern of prosecutors in *Virginia* v. *Webb* (1994) because the defendant made no statement that he intended to kill anyone or that he intended to spread the HIV virus. In the end, the prosecution prevailed, relying in part on a state court of appeals decision holding that specific intent may be shown by circumstances and facts in a particular case.

In *New York* v. *Rios* (1993), a New York Supreme Court judge ruled that a defendant in a drug case who plea-bargained for a reduced sentence and was later determined to be infected with HIV was not entitled to have his plea vacated or sentence set aside. In his decision, the judge rejected the argument that the accused was physically or mentally ill as a result of his seropositivity and therefore "unable to actively participate and comprehend the plea-bargaining meeting." As to the defendant's argument that he was too ill to complete the eighteen-month-to-three-year sentence, the judge cited a State Supreme Court Appellate Division ruling that "It is well settled that affliction with [HIV] or with AIDS, standing alone, does not warrant a reduction in an otherwise appropriate sentence."

In *Applewhite* v. *United States* (1992), a federal appeals court for the District of Columbia ruled that a trial judge had not based her revocation of a convicted burglar's probation on the HIV-infected defendant's possible health threat to the community, adding that even if the court had considered the defendant's health status, "it is by no means clear that such reliance was or would be erroneous." In his pleadings, the appellant, Edgar Applewhite, who had been convicted on two counts of second-degree burglary, argued that in her 1991 decision revoking his probation the trial court judge had improperly concentrated on the fact that he was an HIV-positive drug user. In rejecting appellant's argument, the D.C. Court of Appeals held that the revocation was fully warranted based solely on Applewhite's lengthy history of not complying with probation conditions and missing court hearings. However, the court also held that "if the trial court did rely principally on appellant's HIV-positive status in deciding to revoke his probation, it is by no means clear that such reliance was or would be erroneous. Appellant's medical history has a potentially direct impact on the public health, especially in light of his history of injection drug use." The risk that he might transmit the virus to another drug user or to a sexual partner was substantial, since the court obviously could not guarantee that he would refrain from drug use or sexual activity outside of prison.

Chapter Nine

Worldwide Policies and Practices

In 1987, the World Health Organization (WHO) released the first of several policy statements addressing the prevention and control of HIV and AIDS in the world's prisons (Harding, 1987). These initial guidelines emphasized (1) the necessity of treating all inmates equally regardless of their serostatus, (2) the importance of educating prison staff on HIV and AIDS prevention methods and control issues, and (3) the responsibility of administrators to minimize the transmission of HIV within prison populations. The 1992 recommendations, while similar, are couched in language more specific to particular behaviors which may put inmates at risk for HIV transmission (Schaller, 1993). In this most recent set of guidelines for prison officials, the WHO addresses prevention issues associated with the high incidence of injection drug use and unprotected same-gender sexual acts within prisons. The document states that "even when prohibited, condoms should be available" and "for countries with an increased proportion of drug users in their prison populations, alternative approaches in the management and distribution of disinfectant (e.g., diluted bleach) to prisoners should be taken into consideration" (Schaller, 1993). This chapter addresses prison HIV/AIDS issues across selected foreign countries. Attention is given to HIV testing, risk factors, high-risk sexual activity while incarcerated, injection drug use behavior, and strategies for HIV/AIDS prevention.

Prison administrators worldwide confront high incidences of drug abuse and high-risk sexual activity within their facilities (Thomas & Moerings, 1994). Yet prison staff members are sometimes inadequately educated about HIV and AIDS transmission and prevention issues. Politics and the traditional social mores of each country severely limit the ability of prison officials to implement HIV and AIDS prevention programs, to the detriment of inmates who are more easily infected and prison staff who remain less educated (Thomas & Moerings, 1994).

There is a lack of recognition by the public and some prison administrators regarding the high incidence of some risk behaviors, particularly unprotected same-gender sexual behaviors, among inmates (Thomas & Moerings, 1994). A significant number of countries, such as France, Scotland, and Chile, are willing to acknowledge the existence of injection drug use among inmates. Globally, prison officials wrestle with the moral and ethical issues surrounding needle exchange programs (Feest & Stover, 1994). In some nations, there are concerns that free, sterile equipment would encourage other non-injection drug use inmates to begin experimenting with injection drugs in prison. There is the growing perception among prison officials that in order to halt the spread of HIV in their facilities they must endorse actions contrary to the laws they have sworn to uphold (Feest & Stover, 1994).

A major concern surrounding the transmission of HIV in prisons is the potential for the spread of the virus back into the general population once the inmates have been released (McKee & Power, 1992). Many countries have yet to recognize the threat of HIV transmission in prisons as a problem with viable solutions.

HIV Testing

In countries such as England, Wales, Germany, and Israel, HIV testing upon entrance to prison is a routine service provided to consenting inmates, and it is usually considered voluntary (Turnbull, Dolan, & Stimson, 1993; Dorozynski, 1995; Sheldon, 1995; Karches, 1995; Siegel-Itzkovich, 1995). The definition of *voluntary*, however, seems to vary from country to country and between prison officials and prisoners.

In England and Wales, prisoners are identified by at-risk status for HIV testing (Turnbull et al., 1993). According to ex-inmates who were tested for HIV antibodies, placement in the at-risk category is largely dependent upon sexual orientation and drug use status. Once considered at-risk, inmates are encouraged to take an HIV test; but if they refuse they are placed on viral infectivity restrictions or in isolation until their HIV status can be conclusively determined. One former inmate aptly describes this as follows: "If you get allocated to the bloodtest wing the only way the authorities will treat you as HIV negative is if you get a test. So they are twisting your arm" (Turnbull et al., 1993).

Similar situations exist in German and Israeli prisons. In Bavaria, the only German state where compulsory testing is legal, testing also is carried out on a supposedly voluntary basis. Interviews with German inmates have produced qualitative evidence indicating that the notion of voluntary testing is accompanied by the threat of forced testing (Feest & Stover, 1994). Israeli prisoners are involuntarily tested for HIV. Medical officers in these correctional facilities advocate that all prisoners, without exception, be tested for HIV soon after beginning their incarceration (Siegel-Itzkovich, 1995).

Many inmates refuse the HIV testing available to them upon their arrival in prison (Dorozynski, 1995; Calzavara et al., 1995). In France, it was established that at least 1,620 people out of a total of 57,000 within the penal population were HIV-positive, and 220 of them had developed the clinical symptoms of AIDS (Dorozynski, 1995). However, it is widely assumed that the results of this survey underestimate the actual prevalence of HIV in the French prison population because one in five French prisoners refuses the voluntary and anonymous HIV test (Dorozynski, 1995).

Investigators in many countries believe that those inmates refusing the HIV test may perceive themselves to be at greater risk for infection (Vaz, Gloyd, Folgosa, & Kreiss, 1995). This situation creates a form of selection bias and misrepresents the number of inmates infected with HIV (Calzavara et al., 1995). In Ontario, Canada, investigators carried out a study to reduce volunteer bias in HIV testing using anonymous urine specimens routinely collected from male and female inmates in all Ontario jails from February to August 1993 (Calzavara et al., 1995). Information on sex, age, and history of drug use was matched to each specimen. The overall rates of HIV-1 infection were 1 percent for adult males, 1.2 percent for adult women, and zero percent for young offenders. Rates for HIV-1 infection were found to be highest among self-reported drug users. The results of this study confirm the rate of HIV-1 to be higher among those entering prison than in the general population. Investigators believe that the use of anonymous specimens will be an important tool for measuring actual HIV prevalence rates and will justify much-needed education and health promotion efforts in prisons (Calzavara et al., 1995).

Risk Factors in Prisons

Risk factors for HIV infection among inmates in foreign prisons do not differ greatly from those in the United States. The risk factors include injection drug use, high-risk same-gender sexual behavior, high-risk bisexual sex, high-risk heterosexual sex, low levels of knowledge, and negative attitudes and beliefs surrounding HIV/AIDS. A number of researchers in varying countries have indicated that ex-inmates consider injection drug use to be the greatest risk factor for HIV infection in prison communities. While statistics have supported this assertion, there remains a reluctance to acknowledge the existence of same-gender sex in the prisons. Only now in the mid-1990s are countries recognizing the occurrence of this behavior among inmates. High-risk heterosexual sex has not appeared in the literature as a matter of great concern. A preponderance of the research is clearly focused on drug injection.

High-Risk Sexual Activity

Based on a review of the literature, for some countries the greatest risk factor inmates have for HIV infection is sexual contact. Researchers in Chile, Russia, and Mexico have found evidence to support this claim (Bustos, Arredondo, & Child, 1993; Magis et al., 1994; Albov & Issaev, 1994) found that from 1988 to 1990, the greatest risk behavior for HIV infection among inmates was same-gender and bisexual contact.

England, Wales, Africa, and a number of other countries consider same-gender sexual behavior taboo (Feest & Stover, 1994; Moerings, 1994). England and Wales classify some same-gender sexual acts as criminal offenses under the Sexual Offenses Act of 1967 (Thomas, 1994). The Act states that "a same gender sexual behavior act in private shall not be an offense provided that both parties consent thereto and have attained the age of 21." Due to this law, many gay youths under twenty-one are imprisoned for engaging in behaviors consistent with their sexual orientation. Thomas (1994) found that, at any one time, approximately 20 percent of the English and Welsh prison population is gay men.

It is widely believed that same-gender sexual behavior is uncommon in sub-Saharan Africa (Vaz, Gloyd, Folgosa, & Kreiss, 1995). However, in a cross-sectional study carried out in Mozambique in 1995 among 1,284 male and 54 female prisoners, it was determined that 42 percent ($n = 535$) of males and 20 percent ($n = 11$) of females interviewed believed that sex occurred between same-sex inmates. Seventy (5.5 percent) males and two (4 percent) females reported they had engaged in sexual activity while imprisoned. Of the seventy males, sixty-nine reported that their sexual activities were same-gender in nature. In five gender-segregated prisons in Mozambique, 5 percent of the men interviewed reported same-gender sexual activity. In Zambia, 12.2 percent of the male inmates interviewed also reported sex with other men (Vaz, Gloyd, Folgosa, & Kreiss, 1995).

Internationally, many inmates have reported having had multiple partners and engaging in unprotected sex. Magis et al. (1994) found that HIV infection was mostly associated with sexual relations among men in Mexican prisons. Survey data collected by researchers in Mexican prisons are used to describe the relationship between HIV infection and imprisonment (Magis et al., 1994). In this study, the self-reported sexual risk behaviors of 1,065 male inmates were analyzed. Results of the profile showed that 21.5 percent had sexual relations with only men and 14.3 percent had sexual relations with both men and women.

Albov and Issaev (1994) conducted a study with 1,100 Russian inmates. Eight to ten percent of those surveyed reported engaging in regular same-gender sexual contact as a passive partner. Thirty-three percent of this group participated in oral and anal sex with 30–50 concurrent partners. Two percent of surveyed inmates reported they had engaged in group sex with men while on leave of absence from the prison. Additionally, survey data show that 5–7 percent of the inmates sustained long-term same-gender sexual relationships while in prison. Albov and Issaev (1994) discovered an elite group of inmates possessing their own cadre of male inmates who provided sex only for them. It was subsequently revealed that condoms had not been used in any of these same-gender sexual encounters.

According to The Prison Reform Trust (as cited in Power et al., 1991) Scotland has estimated that 20–30 percent of inmates participate in same-gender sexual acts while incarcerated. Prison guards further inflate this number, reporting that as many as 60 percent of inmates have same-gender sexual contacts within Scottish prisons (as cited in Power et al., 1991a).

In some European countries, such as Austria, Germany, and Belgium, information on same-gender sexual activity is largely unavailable due to the social unacceptability surrounding such behavior (Feest & Stover, 1994; De Wit, 1994; Pont, Strutz, Kahl, & Salzner, 1994). Some researchers have indicated that this lack of information may be indicative of the level of same-gender sexual activity in different prisons (McKee & Power, 1992). They maintain that cultural taboos and "macho man" ethics may significantly decrease the impulse to engage in same-gender sexual activities (McKee & Power, 1992; Platek, 1994).

Injection Drug Use

Researchers from France have reported injection drug use as the greatest risk factor for HIV infection within their prisons (Rotily et al., 1994; Power et al., 1994; Bustos et al., 1993). A study of inmates in southeastern French prisons revealed a high prevalence of HIV infection, particularly among injection drug users. Of the 432 study participants, 84 (20 percent) were heroin users. Of those, 51 percent reported that they had shared needles prior to being incarcerated, 23 percent indicated they had had more than two sexual partners during the last year, and 13 percent had engaged in sexual intercourse with someone who was HIV-positive in the last five years (Rotily et al., 1994).

Similar results were found by researchers who examined self-perceived risk of HIV infection among inmates inside and outside Scottish prisons (Power et al., 1991a). Five hundred fifty-nine inmates in Scottish prisons were asked to assess their self-perceived risk for HIV infection prior to incarceration. Investigators found that those whose self-perceived risk was greatest were more likely to have been previously charged and sentenced with a drug offense, injected drugs, shared needles inside and outside of prison, had the HIV antibody test, known someone who had been tested, known someone diagnosed HIV-positive, had sexual contact with an injection drug user, and had more than one sexual partner during the month prior to their incarceration.

In Chile, injection drug use did not present itself as a major risk factor for inmates until 1992 (Bustos et al., 1993). In 1991, five out of twenty-two HIV-positive inmates were injection drug users; in 1992, seven out of twenty-nine HIV-positive inmates were injection drug users (Bustos et al., 1993).

Other risk factors include low levels of HIV knowledge and negative attitudes toward HIV/AIDS. A survey on the knowledge of and attitudes of military recruits and inmates toward HIV/AIDS was conducted in Hungary. Gerlel, Szlavik, Banhegyi, and Miskovits (1994) distributed anonymous surveys to recruits and inmates. Eighty-six percent ($n = 620$) of the inmates responded. Five percent of respondents reported same-gender sexual contact and 2.5 percent reported injection drug use at least once in their life. Sixty percent of those who answered the survey were fearful of contracting HIV. Fifty percent did not believe that they were at risk or thought they were at low risk for infection. Twenty-five percent of the inmates in the Hungarian prison had never heard of AIDS, and only 25 percent had correct knowledge on how HIV is transmitted (Gerlel et al., 1994).

In prisons, the percentage of persons belonging to the high-risk group of injection drug users is higher than that of the general population. In Austria, this is explained by the fact that under current law a high percentage of injection drug users spend time in prison (Pont et al., 1994).

Strategies for HIV/AIDS Prevention

Prevention activities in prisons throughout the world are varied in nature, but they usually focus on creating safer climates for drug-addicted inmates and those engaging in high-risk sexual activity. Many investigators have stressed the need for education, citing that prisons provide an unparalleled opportunity to "inform and educate large numbers of persons who have engaged or may be likely to engage in [high risk] behaviors" (Vaz, Gloyd, Folgosa, & Kreiss, 1995). Unfortunately, many inmates do not have access to the same services as noninmates, such as needle exchange and condom distribution programs. This lack of services can be attributed to bans on drugs, needles, and syringes in some prisons (Platek, 1994; Feest & Stover, 1994) and the perception by some correctional authorities that same-gender sexual behavior is virtually nonexistent (Mudur, 1995). In addition to the belief that same-gender sexual behavior does not exist, in some countries there are also legal issues surrounding the distribution of condoms. India, for example, cites same-gender sexual behavior as an offense under the Indian Penal Code of 1860. Any programs designed to provide condoms to inmates would be perceived as "aiding and abetting" this crime (Mudur, 1995).

However, many prisons in European countries do offer condoms to their inmates (Scherdin, 1994; Pont et al., 1994; Feest & Stover, 1994; Taylor et al., 1995; Dolley, 1995; Dorozynski, 1995). In 1989, the incoming Christian Democrat Minister of Justice in Belgium, Melchior Wathelet, distributed a letter to prison officials providing for the purchase of condoms in prison canteens throughout the country (De Wit, 1994).

Switzerland is currently providing both condoms and needle exchange programs to its inmates (Dorozynski, 1995). In 1994, a pilot project was initiated to begin the distribution of sterile injection equipment to female inmates (Bernasconi, Buechi, & Stutz, 1994). A pilot project was created to introduce preventive measures for HIV transmission. The intent of the project was to provide the female inmates with sterile injecting equipment and ensure access to the same preventive measures outside the prison system. This particular project emphasizes in-service training for the prison staff and acknowledgment of the special needs of female inmates (Bernasconi et al., 1994).

Many countries are focusing their prevention activities on both inmates and staff. De Jongh-Wieth and Schepp-Beelen (1994) have identified ways of promoting safer sex practices and provide care and support to inmates in the Netherlands. Collaboration between prison, rehabilitation, and public health personnel has resulted in a nonjudgmental, nonmoralizing attitude by prison staff, and a safe climate for inmates to seek counseling (de Jongh-Wieth & Schepp-Beelen, 1994).

Research by Jurgens, Gilmore, and Richard (1993) shows similar procedures have been adopted in Canada. Input from inmates concerning availability of condoms, bleach and clean needles/syringes, education about HIV/AIDS, drug use, confidentiality, and testing has been solicited by prison officials. Prison staff have also been polled about their personal concerns and opinions regarding HIV/AIDS, drug use in prisons, and ideas to promote a safe working environment.

In Australia, prison officials have implemented policies and programs designed to minimize the transmission of HIV in prisons. Strategies introduced in Australian prisons include bleach availability, HIV antibody testing, education for staff, peer education for the inmates, a unit for HIV-infected inmates, specialized videos, and AIDS committees and awareness days (Vumbaca, 1994). To date, the results of this intervention have been positive. In the last eighteen months, fewer than five inmates have seroconverted while in prison. A number of inmates have also shown increases in knowledge and level of awareness and a reduction in prejudices toward those who are HIV-positive (Vumbaca, 1994).

Similar interventions have been instituted in Scottish prisons. Emslie, Taylor, Goldberg, Wrench, and Gruer (1994) describe projects that include a public health initiative designed to educate inmates. Consenting inmates are tested for HIV, counseled about risk behaviors which facilitate the transmission of blood-borne infections, and educated about measures which could prevent further infection through counseling and testing (Emslie et al., 1994).

Oliveira and Longo (1993) report findings concerning Projeto Tereza in Brazil. Projeto Tereza is designed to emphasize the risk of sexual transmission of HIV within prisons in Rio de Janeiro. Its goal is to encourage inmates to reflect on their sexuality and associated high-risk behaviors. Methods used include a study of existing projects worldwide, personal interviews with 2,300 inmates in Rio de Janeiro, and an evaluation of the impact of educational materials on inmates. Because 73 percent of the inmates in Rio reported engaging in same-gender sexual activities, the most effective means for decreasing the incidence of high-risk sexual behaviors has been the distribution of materials demonstrating safer sex practices and the promotion of an open relationship with the educator (Oliveira & Longo, 1993).

Conclusion

The debate surrounding prisons and HIV/AIDS seems to focus consistently on the distribution of condoms and sterile injecting equipment. It is evident that other critical factors should be considered. The prison environment and culture should be responsive to the needs of both staff and inmates. Any efforts at education should emphasize a positive, consistent relationship between the educator and the inmate.

Prison officials must consider the strong cultural taboo against same-gender sex in some prisons. Based on the large number of inmates who indicate participation in same-gender sex activities, it must be emphasized in education. The primary association of HIV with drug use demonstrates a strong prejudice and ignores other high-risk behaviors. Each prison system throughout the world must take steps to deal with the increasing incidence of HIV in a socially responsible and appropriate manner.

Chapter Ten

The Public Health Challenge

There is an enormous personal, familial, and public health price to pay for treatment intervention after the onset of HIV/AIDS. This realization may account for the considerable increase in attention and support for HIV prevention programs directed toward reducing the damage being done in our society by risky sexual behavior and illicit drug use. This book amplifies the challenges involved in designing and deploying effective HIV prevention strategies to confront self-destructive drug use and sexual behaviors among prison and jail inmates. In any effective prevention program, there is a need for the target population to define the problem and participate in the assessment phase, prior to implementation of an intervention. In this context, *prevention* is taken to mean not necessarily the complete elimination of the problem but rather a significant reduction of harm (Room, 1974). Additionally, we must closely monitor the costs and benefits that are likely to ensue. With many infectious diseases, rehabilitation is plausible; but HIV/AIDS usually involves coping, while the infected endure anguish over the debilitating and eventually fatal nature of the disease.

Inmates represent a marginalized population—to many, an invisible population since to be out of sight is to be out of mind. Once inmates are convicted and sentenced to the correctional system, their debt to society often translates into simply serving time. For many inmates, the prison experience provides an opportunity to become more criminally sophisticated. For those who are not rehabilitated, it is a chance to acquire new skills and build the capacity for executing new crimes against persons and property. A parallelism exists for those incarcerated who fail to be educated to change risky sexual behavior and illicit drug use prior to release. Prison also represents an opportunity to engage in risky behaviors. A major public health challenge lies in the release of inmates from prison who continue to practice risky behaviors habituated by injection drug use, needle sharing, and unprotected sex.

As indicated in Chapter Five, only two state prison systems (Vermont and Mississippi) and four city/county jail systems (New York City, Philadelphia, San Francisco, and Washington, DC) reported making condoms available to inmates in their facilities. Of the eighty prison and jail systems participating in the 1994 NIJ/CDC survey, only one city/county jail system reported making bleach available to inmates to clean their "works." Many correctional administrators reject these policies, arguing that they would encourage illegal behavior prohibited by correctional regulations as well as state and federal laws. The evidence, however, points to a different reality: effective prevention programs must include practical risk-reduction strategies and approaches with a known high potential of success in HIV prevention. Clearly, the promotion of condoms and cleaning of injection material, for example, must be objectively considered in light of behaviors known to occur in the prison setting. Less than fifteen years ago, these same beliefs plagued public school systems during the sharp debate over the appropriateness of sex education and family life education programs as school activities. However, with the advent of the AIDS crisis, local school boards have grown to accept the need for grade-level and developmentally appropriate early intervention with family life and human growth and development content in the school curriculum. An important challenge to the public health field is to convince correctional officials that a harm-reduction approach to HIV prevention can be consistent with institutional security.

A climate of suspicion and mistrust often exists among corrections agencies, public health agencies, and community-based organizations (CBOs). They often mistrust and misconstrue the others' agendas and intentions, making collaboration difficult if not impossible. For example, corrections agencies may believe that public health professionals are liberals intent only on getting condoms and clean needles into prisons, with no regard for the security and discipline issues that may be involved. Conversely, public health personnel may view correctional personnel as uniformly reactionary people concerned only about security and having no interest in inmates' health. CBOs often mistrust all government agencies, believing that they are not fully committed to the struggle against AIDS. As a starting point for overcoming these barriers to collaboration (and to more cost-efficient as well as effective approaches to HIV prevention in correctional facilities), what is important is more opportunity for honest and open dialogue. For example, conferences and meetings that bring together corrections, public health, and CBO staff may provide the opportunity for increased dissemination of information on successful collaborations as a desirable activity. Too often, these organizations meet only with their own kind, the outcome being esoteric discussion and thus perpetuation of mistrust and misinformation across these systems.

Public health agencies at all levels should foster and initiate interagency agreements and collaborations with adult correctional systems, juvenile justice systems, and CBOs to develop responsive HIV/AIDS education and prevention programs in prisons, jails, and juvenile facilities. Moreover, given the eventual release of almost all adult inmates and confined juveniles to the community, it is incumbent upon health and human service systems to become proactive rather than reactive in planning for the reintegration of these populations back into the community. This will require the establishment of effective coalitions and partnerships between these systems to promote and help sustain risk reduction among the uninfected and those still engaging in risky behaviors. With this foregoing sketch as a backdrop to the complexities of the problem, the following specific challenges to the public health community are presented.

A Call for Action

Collaboration

Public health professionals should collaborate with correctional administrators to formulate and implement policy regarding HIV/AIDS education and prevention programs in prisons, jails, and juvenile facilities. This will mean a new and nontraditional type of outreach for state health departments and local health department personnel. Such agencies have generally limited their scope of interventions to noninstitutionalized members of society. Collaboration will also mean a new role for correctional administrators who have security as their primary mission. This type of newly forged partnership will fortify the rehabilitation mission of correctional institutions.

Much like the work done in community mental health with the deinstitutionalization of the mentally ill and the use of halfway houses and other transitional facilities, public health professionals will need to work with community-based facilities to facilitate the continuum of reinforcement of HIV/AIDS education and prevention activities. This means that local and state public health assistance will be required by group homes, prerelease centers, and other transitional housing facilities to buttress the prevention message. Because there is no "magic bullet," inmates and ex-offenders will need reinforcement at every juncture until the message is effectively conveyed that risky behaviors are life threatening to themselves and others. This message needs to be accompanied by other support systems that assist this population with counseling, testing, comprehensive and credible programs of interactive education, partner notification, and practical risk-reduction techniques (safer sex and safer drug injection).

Broadening of Attitudes

Another important challenge to public health is the general attitude that inmate populations deserve no special attention or allocation of limited prevention funds. Such a narrow perspective ignores the reality that the vast majority of inmates return to the community upon release; thus, the potential problem is no longer limited to prisons. Whether the prevention effort is focused in prison or on the parolee, it is done for the common good.

Given the high rates of recidivism among both adults and juveniles, it becomes imperative that correctional administrators have formal agreements with public health agencies to facilitate partner notification for known HIV-seropositive cases. This will involve outreach to the families and significant others of the inmate popula-

tion. This will also involve a case-finding role for such health practitioners. Finding partners for notification of potential infection is
difficult enough for the nonincarcerated, and it becomes even
more entangled for the high-risk incarcerated persons, who may
have had partners with whom they have little-to-no identifying
information.

The Federal Response

There is also a challenge regarding the response of the U.S. Public Health Service to the HIV/AIDS crisis, and claims of uncoordinated efforts among federal departments. This charge of
uncoordinated delivery of services for the HIV-infected will require
a new sense of collaborative federal leadership, to be provided by
the White House Office on AIDS; the CDC; and Justice, HRSA, and
other federal departments. These departments must require the
enforcement of laws and policies designed to protect the civil
rights of citizens likely to be discriminated against because of HIV-
positive status. Correctional and public health officials should consider the Americans with Disabilities Act as potential legislative
mandates for achieving equity for the HIV-infected. The need for
monitoring by federal, state, and "watchdog" groups to safeguard
the rights of at-risk and HIV-infected ex-offenders and other citizens becomes apparent in considering issues connected with private health insurance companies (access to health insurance for
employees who work for small companies), hospitals (refusing to
treat HIV-infected patients), pharmaceutical companies (prohibi-
tive costs for certain drugs used in treating HIV/AIDS), schools
(admission and attendance policies), and employers (hiring and
termination policies).

Recognition of the Sterile-Needle Issue

Given that one-third of all AIDS cases reported to CDC are directly
or indirectly related to injection drug use, public health practitioners need to become involved with policymakers from law,
boards of pharmacy, ethics, medicine, and substance abuse as they
deliberate on sensitive issues pertinent to the emerging syringe
laws. The multiperson use (sharing) of injection equipment, particularly needles and syringes, is the major mechanism through

which HIV infection is transmitted from one injection drug user to another. The National Academy of Sciences (Normand, Vlahov, & Moses, 1995) reported that for injection drug users who cannot or will not stop injecting drugs, the once-only use of sterile needles and syringes remains the safest, most-effective approach for limiting HIV transmission. While some states require a physician's prescription to purchase syringes, in other states there is no prescription law. Public health professionals need to become involved in policy formulation pertinent to the sale, distribution, and possession of sterile syringes. From a harm-reduction perspective, these are difficult and challenging issues for public health and correctional policy makers.

Access to Condoms

There is a major myth in the African American community that black males are sent to prison in large numbers to contract HIV. To some, prisons are seen as breeding grounds for the virus, and sexual relations (by consent or force) is the mode of transmission. What is interesting about this conspiracy theory is that it has not prevented sexual contact among inmates, and penal institutions typically do not distribute condoms. The belief that AIDS is a form of genocide is rooted in a social context in which African Americans, faced with persistent inequality, believe in conspiracy theories about whites against African Americans (Thomas & Quinn, 1991). One way that policymakers can win back the trust and overcome some of the myths that hinder HIV prevention in these settings is to provide inmates with access to condoms. While such a proposal may be controversial, it remains a viable public health option to reduce the spread of HIV.

Increased Testing and Counseling

Public health professionals and policy makers should also consider forming collaborative relationships with state and federal probation and parole boards to address issues such as criteria for HIV testing of parolees and probationers. More widely available HIV counseling and testing programs may be vehicles for reaching more parolees and probationers with counseling and referral services.

Social Communicative Factors

For prevention efforts to be successful among this population, public health researchers need to evaluate social interactions in correctional institutions among prisoners and the penal staff (correctional officers, health staff, and others). Evaluation of the dynamics of these interactions, in conjunction with sexual relationships and their primary determinants in prison populations, should be systematically conducted, including the use of ethnographic methods since communication may be altered by artifacts of interpersonal communication, such as fear, survival impulses, and/or a type of learned helplessness.

Prisoners (especially males) may feel that contemplating healthy lifestyles is not plausible in jail. Thus, the level of preventive efforts should be based on length of sentence and the social-cultural experiences of the inmate. For example, individuals serving short sentences may be more responsive to messages that are directed toward minimizing contact with body fluids of others; the messages could result in less physical assaults if they are presented in an acceptable manner that some inmates respect. Perhaps this could be done by known gang leaders. Having Muslims serve as prevention messengers may be another avenue for reaching youthful African Americans, given the Muslims' reputation of success in dissuading youths from drug use.

There also exists an enormous public health challenge for addressing the needs of female inmates. There are serious gaps in provision of routine gynecological screening and care for female inmates, as well as shortfalls in prenatal and perinatal care for pregnant females in prisons and jails. These services are clearly key elements of a comprehensive HIV/AIDS prevention and treatment program for incarcerated women. In addition, the constellation of problems faced by many drug-involved women who find themselves in prisons and jails—abusive sexual relationships, loss of custody of children, involvement in commercial sex work, generally stressful and chaotic lives—suggests the challenges and opportunities for providing practical, culturally appropriate, and ultimately effective HIV prevention programs to incarcerated women. Public health agencies and CBOs have much to contribute to this important effort.

Education and Prevention Programs for Juveniles

Public health professionals, in conjunction with correctional personnel, need to generate and field test HIV/AIDS education and prevention programs designed for juvenile offenders in a cultural context. Such prevention programs will require significant input from juveniles; social marketing principles should be employed to maximize acceptability. Focus groups have been one useful strategy for testing acceptability to various markets. We believe that creative expression through such modes as rap songs, dance, theater, videography, and photo-novellas or comic books, generated and delivered by peer leaders, will increase this population's receptivity to HIV prevention messages. This type of intervention represents a challenge to the public health agencies, but it would seem to be advanced by collaboration with professionals from the humanities. ·

Professional Preparation

Another critical challenge to public health educators relates to the need for schools of public health to assess the extent to which their curricula effectively prepare their graduates to engage and work with communities (particularly disenfranchised communities) and CBOs on HIV/AIDS and a host of other health issues. Community organization and development (COD) for health-promotion and disease-prevention programming are essential skill areas for public health students planning to work in populations with disproportionate rates of morbidity and mortality. Implementing student practicum and internship experiences within correctional facilities represents a promising new initiative for public health educators. This challenge can be addressed through academic self-study and establishing correctional practicum experiences and course work focused on COD principles. Such course content has its roots in curricula at schools of social work; it represents another discipline in which public health educators can seek collaboration.

In summary, one might ask whose responsibility it is to address the need for HIV/AIDS prevention among inmates. We are reminded of the story involving four people named Everybody, Somebody,

Anybody, and Nobody. There was an important job to be done; Everybody knew that Somebody would do it, and that Anybody could do it; but Nobody did it. Somebody got angry because he knew it was Everybody's job. Everybody knew that Anybody could do it, but Nobody realized that Everybody would not do it. So, in the end, Everybody blamed Somebody when Nobody did what Anybody could have done.

We can all play a role in meeting the public health challenge of HIV/AIDS among adult and juvenile offenders. We only need the will and commitment to do the job.

Afterword

Once characterized as a disease of men who engaged in same-gender sexual contact, HIV/AIDS is fast becoming an inner-city, multigenerational, family disease. The growing importance of the institutional context in the AIDS epidemic is vividly illustrated in this book, *Prisons and AIDS: A Public Health Challenge.* Authors Braithwaite, Hammett, and Mayberry have done the field an important service by describing how various types of jails and prisons provide a cauldron for dangerous and risky behaviors that contribute to high rates of HIV infection and AIDS. What I found especially important about the book is the authors' essential point that prison institutions are linked to other institutions, such as the family and the community. Thus prisons pose a significant public health threat by increasing substantially the already serious problems of HIV infection that face individuals and families that reside in areas of concentrated poverty and high criminal activity.

Using demographic, epidemiological, and national survey data, the authors illuminate the scope of the problem prisons pose and the inadequate response at all levels of government. While acknowledging the political difficulties in implementing programs such as bleach and condom distribution in prisons, the authors point out the need for public health interventions to reduce the potential threat of creating institutions that are a breeding ground for the disease. All over this country and across the globe, a growing emphasis is being placed on punishment and incarceration in response to crime. Because those who are likely to be punished and incarcerated are drawn from populations likely to engage in high-risk behaviors, there is the potential for the spread of the disease to others within prisons. Because those in prison are more likely than not released back into their former communities, there is the opportunity for continued infection and the introduction of the virus into the unsuspecting community.

The authors have provided an even-handed account of the problem, but I want to point to the special threat AIDS poses to ethnic minority individuals in prisons. In Michigan, for example, it has been reported that over 50 percent of inmates are African American, although the African American population is no more than 15 percent of the total state population. The high concentration of the African American and Latino populations in neighborhoods with high poverty, poor employment opportunities, and high drug traffic provides for the disproportionate risk of arrest and imprisonment. Because of these facts, it is clear that at every turn, minority men, women, and adolescents are at greater risk than Americans of European background for exposure to and contracting of HIV and AIDS.

Because of the nature of the risks of exposure to the HIV virus and its spread, social psychological processes and social behavior are prime targets of concern. We know that social and economic circumstances can contribute to greater risk of contracting HIV, independent of ethnic status. It is also clear that cultural patterns—independent of socioeconomic and ethnic status—can contribute to greater exposure and reduced efficacy of social and behavioral interventions designed to reduce risk and behavioral and medical interventions designed to extend life.

Finally, both legal and illegal immigration, younger age distrubtions, higher birth rates among minority populations, and the continuing pattern of geographical discrimination will contribute to the growth for several decades of culturally and linguistically diverse groups. These populations will be either unacculturated or, like African Americans, systematically excluded from mainstream social, economic, and cultural institutions in the United States. These groups will be prime candidates for disproportionate arrests and incarceration. Complex interactions among these social, economic, and ethnic factors and their relationship to sexual, drug-related, and other risk behaviors tied to HIV infection and AIDS must be understood if we are to develop and mount effective interventions and treatment strategies in African American and diverse ethnic populations. The fact that imprisonment will figure so prominently in the lives of members of these groups is problematic.

Prisons and AIDS is a hopeful book predicated on the need for a proactive public health orientation to the problem. The fact is that prisons provide a level of social organization and potential control that is absent in the larger society. It is possible—even with the current high rates of seropositive individuals in prisons—that much can be done to effectively intervene using known and tested public health methods. In the last chapter of the book, the authors focus on some of these potential public health interventions. These include developing a realistic understanding of the nature of the problem. The authors point out, rightly so, that political attitudes about prisons make it difficult to implement many public health programs. This has to change. As the incarcerated population increases—and the proportion of seropositive individuals increases as well—it is clear that something must be done.

The authors note how the problem differs between male and female prison populations. Among females, the lack of routine gynecological care and prenatal and perinatal care for pregnant inmates is a serious problem. There may be a need to get inmate organizations and external culturally specific organizations—such as the Black Muslims—more involved in the development of educational and behavioral intervention programs. Special attention may need to be placed on juvenile facilities where the growing rate of STDs serves as a barometer of a coming crisis. Finally, the authors point to the need for better education of public health officials and workers in the special needs of prison institutions. More and better training will be required to develop effective, knowledgeable, and experienced public health professionals. Certainly the current low level of programs and small number of professionals trained to address these issues are woefully inadequate.

At the end of the book, Braithwaite, Hammett, and Mayberry point to the conundrum of the *Everybody, Somebody, Anybody, and Nobody* problem. By documenting the national and international scope of the problem of HIV and AIDS in prisons, the woefully inadequate public health response, and the danger and risks to the society at large, the book unequivocally testifies to the fact that this disease is *Everybody's* problem.

July 1996   JAMES S. JACKSON
Daniel Katz Distinguished University Professor of Psychology
Director and Research Scientist
Program for Research on Black Americans
Institute for Social Research
University of Michigan

A Guide to Education and Prevention Resources

There exist a wide range of useful HIV/AIDS education and prevention resources in the public domain. This chapter is intended as a resource guide for those working with incarcerated social offenders. The materials herein are not exhaustive, but rather designed to identify pertinent resources to be used across correctional populations. The curriculum and audiovisual materials referenced herein have been screened for relevance and accuracy of information. We encourage those working with incarcerated populations to incorporate educational resources that are not specific to the correctional population (general HIV/AIDS resources), since much of this information has utility across at-risk populations.

We encourage you to contact the resources identified in this chapter if you desire to identify materials that have been used within correctional settings. In this guide you will find

1. A list of HIV/AIDS advocacy organizations that have worked among or on behalf of correctional populations
2. HIV/AIDS prevention and educational audiovisual resources
3. Curriculum materials
4. Related HIV/AIDS publications that have been used with this population

HIV/AIDS Inmate Advocacy Organizations

ACE Out
103 East 125th St., Suite 602
New York, NY 10035
(212) 673–6633
Peer support, counseling, referrals for HIV-positive men on parole.

ACLU National Prison Project
1875 Connecticut Ave. N.W., Suite 410
Washington, DC 20009
(202) 234–4830 attn.: Jackie Walker
Information, advocacy, referrals, support for peer education projects.

ACT UP/San Francisco Prison Issues Committee
P.O. Box 14844
San Francisco, CA 94114
(415) 522–2907

AIDS in Prison Project
135 East 15th St.
New York, NY 10003
Hotline (212) 674–0800 attn.: The Osborne Association
Information, referrals, advocacy; accepts collect calls from prisoners on Tuesdays/Thursdays from 3:00 to 8:00 P.M.

AIDS Legal Referral Panel
Box 1983
San Francisco, CA 94101
(415) 864–5156
Legal help for persons with AIDS or ARC either at reduced cost or for free.

AIDS Prison Initiative/Rural Opportunities, Inc.
140 N. Main St.
Albion, NY 14411
(716) 589–7027 attn.: John Till or Catalina Montes
(800) 365–7027 service line
Peer education, support groups, HIV counseling and testing, referrals for parole for women at Albion Correctional Facility.

AIDS/HIV in Correctional Settings
U.S. Conference of Mayors
1620 Eye St., N.W.
Washington, DC 20006
(202) 293–7330

ALIANA
P.O. Box 53396
Washington, DC 20009
Information about AIDS. A project of the Latin-American community.

American Red Cross Statewide HIV/AIDS Education/Network
Coordinators
81111 Gatehouse Rd.
Falls Church, VA 22042
(703) 206–7180 attn.: Kristine Ripley

The Body Positive
19 Fulton St., Suite 3038B
New York, NY 10038
(212) 566–7333
Information for HIV-positive people.

Center for Community Alternatives
39 West 19th St., 3rd Floor
New York, NY 10011
(212) 691–1911
AIDS/HIV-related prevention and support services to inmates, parolees, and their families.

The Correctional HIV Consortium
3463 State St., #204
Santa Barbara, CA 93105
(805) 568–1400 or (805) 899–3820
This organization provides assistance in meeting the challenge of HIV disease within the criminal justice system and corrections communities.

Correctional Services Program
30th St. and Walnut
Kansas City, MO 64108

Fortune Society
39 West 19th St.
New York, NY 10011
(212) 206–7070 attn.: D. Dawood
Management, advocacy, referrals, support, AIDS and drug use
information.

Gay American Indians AIDS Project
333 Valencia St. #207
San Francisco, CA 94103
AIDS awareness and prevention program; services for Native Americans with AIDS/ARC/HIV.

HIV/AIDS in Prison Project of Catholic Charities
433 Jefferson St.
San Francisco, CA 94607
(510) 834–5656
Impacts public policy concerning the care and treatment of prisoners with HIV and AIDS; community education.

Howard University National AIDS Minority Information
2139 Georgia Ave. N.W., Suite 3-B
Washington, DC 20001
(202) 865–3720
Peggy Valentine, Ed.D., project director

Intercouncil Community Fellowship
60 West 130th St., #1A
New York, NY 10037
(212) 722-AIDS or (212) 722–8695
Case management, support groups, education, referral, etc., for
women of color with AIDS/HIV, incarcerated or recently released.

Intertribal Council of Arizona, Inc.
4205 North 7th Ave., Suite 200
Phoenix, AZ 85013
(602) 248–0071
John R. Lewis, executive director

KITE
The Correctional HIV Consortium, Inc.
3463 State St. #204
Santa Barbara, CA 93105
(805) 568–1400
Monthly publication.

Legal AIDS Society, Prisoner's Rights Project
15 Park Row, 7th Floor
New York, NY 10038
(212) 577–3530 attn.: Jack Beck or Michael Wiesman
Provides legal advocacy to prisoners.

National Alliance of State and Territorial AIDS Directors
444 N. Capitol St. N.W., Suite 706
Washington, DC 20001
(202) 434–8090

National Commission of Correctional Health Care
2105 N. Southport, Suite 200
Chicago, IL 60614
(312) 528-0818

National Institute of Justice
1600 Research Blvd.
Rockville, MD 20880
Publications.

National Latino/a Lesbian and Gay Organization (LLEGO)
703 G St., S.E.
Washington, DC 20003
(202) 544–0092
Letitia Gomez, executive director

National Lawyers Guild AIDS Network
55a Capp St.
San Francisco, CA 94110
(415) 285-5067

National Minority AIDS Council (NMAC)
300 I St. N.E., Suite 400
Washington, DC 20002
(202) 544-1076
Paul Kawata, executive director

The National Native American AIDS Prevention Center
(NNAAPC)
3515 Grand Ave., Suite 100
Oakland CA 94610
(510) 444-2051
Ron Rowell, executive director

National Prison Hospice Association
P.O. Box 55
Boulder, CO 80306-0058
Assists in development of hospice/palliative care programs for
dying prisoners and their families.

National Prison Project
1875 Connecticut Ave., NE, Suite 410
Washington, DC 20009

National Task Force on AIDS Prevention
631 O'Farrell St.
San Francisco, CA 94109
(415) 749-6700
Randy Miller, executive director

Northwest Portland Area Indian Health Board
520 S.W. Harrison, Suite 440
Portland, OR 97201
(503) 228-4185
Doni Wilder, executive director

Nutrition Information for People with AIDS and ARC
Dept. of Public Health
101 Grove St., Room 118
San Francisco, CA 94102
(415) 554-2500

P.A.C.E. Green Haven
Green Haven Correctional Facility
Drawer B
Stormville, NY 12582
(914) 221–2711
Richard Stanulwich, staff advisor

People with AIDS Coalition Newsline
31 West 26th St.
New York, NY 10011
(212) 647–1415
Monthly newsletter free to people with AIDS; free pen pal listing.

Prison AIDS Resource Center
P.O. Box 2155
Vacaville, CA 95696–8155
Information and support.

Prison Book Program
92 Green St.
Jamaica Plain, MA 02130

Prisoners Legal Services of New York
105 Chambers St., 2nd Floor
New York, NY 10077
(212) 513–7373 attn.: David Leven
Provides legal services to indigent inmates in NYS prisons.

Prisoners with AIDS Rights Advocacy Group (PWA RAG)
P.O. Box 216
Jonesboro, GA 30237
(770) 946–9346
Information and support, free quarterly newsletter, advocacy.

Professional Organizations National Commission on Correctional
Health Care
2105 N. Southport, Suite 200
Chicago, IL 60614
(312) 528–0818

Puerto Rican Organization for Community Education and Economic Development, Inc. (PROCEED)
815 Elizabeth Ave.
Elizabeth, NJ 07201
(908) 351–7727 attn.: Heriberto Sanchez-Soto
A nonprofit organization that provides services to the local community, such as rental, food, health, AIDS education, and substance abuse programs, as well as a youth center and a daycare center.

PWA Prison Project
P.O. Box 300339
Denver, CO 80203
Organizes and educates around prison issues, for prisoners and corrections staff.

The Sentencing Project
918 F St. N.W., Suite 501
Washington, DC 20004
(202) 628–0871
Provides information concerning current topics in corrections.

Stand Up Harlem
145 West 130th St.
New York, NY 10027
(212) 926–4072
Housing and support services for people with AIDS/HIV released from prison; prison ministry.

United Migrant Opportunity Services, Inc. (UMOS)
929 West Mitchell St.
Milwaukee, WI 53204
(414) 671–5700
Mary Ann Borman, project director
UMOS provides social services to the migrant population.

U.S. Mexico Border Health Association (USMBHA)
6006 N. Mesa, Suite 600
El Paso, TX 79912
(915) 581–6645
Rebeca Ramos, project director
Created in 1943 to provide health services to the cities along the
U.S. and Mexico border.

Women's Prison Association (WPA)
110 Second Ave.
New York, NY 10003
(212) 674–1163
Serves Bedford Hills and Taconic prisons. WPA provides shelter to
incarcerated women with open court dates. It also provides workshops and day programs.

List of HIV/AIDS Audiovisual Materials

A Bad Way to Die
Taconic Correctional Facility
250 Harris Rd.
Bedford Hills, NY 10507
Video targeting prison populations.

A First Step: AIDS Prevention for Drug Abusers
State of New York Department of Health, AIDS Institute
1215 Western Ave., Suite 306
Albany, NY 12203
(518) 431–1218 attn.: Tracy McCumber
This video includes a demonstration of cleaning syringes with
bleach to kill the HIV virus.

A Will to Live
SBG Productions
2724 Dorr Ave.
Fairfax, VA 22031
(703) 698–7750
This video is available in both male and female versions.

AIDS Is About Secrets
The HIV Center
722 West 188th St.
New York, NY 10032
(212) 740–0047 attn.: Kenia Fernandez
Video for African American women who are partners of injection drug users.

Audio Visual Unit
New York City Department of Correction Academy
66–26 Metropolitan Ave.
Middle Village, NY 11379
Peer support, counseling, referrals for HIV-positive women on parole. Titles include *Recovery Is an Inside Job, Word from the Joint, Doing Life and Living with AIDS, A Hospice for Us, Women Get AIDS Too, Plain Talk About Tattoos, Shoot Clean, Condoms for Cons, How Do I Know You're Okay?, Don't Take an Unwanted Gift on Parole.*

Breaking the Silence
The HIV Center
722 West 188th St.
New York, NY 100032
(212) 740–0047 attn.: Kenia Fernandez
AIDS prevention video for Hispanic women; available in both English and Spanish.

Brother Earl
Department of Corrections, Office of Substance Abuse Programs
Video Loan Library
524 I St.
Sacramento, CA 95814
(916) 327–3707 attn.: Rita A. Norman

Color Me Clean: Black Women in Recovery
Black Eyes Productions
Two parts, 30 minutes each. Four black women—Joy, Debra, Jill and Brenda—tell and relive their experiences with drug addiction. Their contrasting stories move the viewer and highlight issues unique to black women in recovery. An extremely candid and engrossing program. Call Number: Vid 20/20.1.

Con-to-Con
Positive Life With HIV
190 Fifth St. East, Suite 200
Saint Paul, MN 55101–1637
(612) 225–9035; fax (612) 225–9102
Independent Television Service (ITVS) video.

The Correctional HIV Consortium Corporate Headquarters
150 Francisco Street, #216
San Francisco, CA 93105
(800) 572–9310
Audiovisual lending library of more than 200 titles, mostly of general HIV/AIDS subjects. A number of these deal with substance use, and other issues relevant to prisoners and prison/correctional populations.

Crack Cocaine
Pride, Inc.
3610 Dekalb Technology Pkwy., Suite 105
Atlanta, GA 30340
(770) 458–9900
Instructional media, nine one-hour videos plus a 300-page curriculum and instructor's manual. English and Spanish. This personal video was developed to present the impact of crack cocaine on the human mind and body. The target viewer may be in a jail cell, a treatment center or prison, or a member of the community simply wanting to learn more about the most dangerous drug of the nineties. Call Number: Vid 24.

Department of Corrections
Office of Substance Abuse Programs
524 I St.
Sacramento, CA 95814
(916) 327–3707 attn.: Rita A. Norman

Free Your Mind
Office of Substance Abuse Programs
524 I St.
Sacramento, CA 95814
(916) 327–3707 attn.: Rita A. Norman

Series of videos: (1) *Perceptions and Priorities,* 19 minutes; (2) *Choices and Consequences,* 40 minutes; (3) *Abstinence, Awareness, Choice, and Change,* 16 minutes; (4) *From Chains to Change,* 51 minutes. This series, focusing on common-sense delivery by ex-offenders with years of crime-free living and successful reintegration into society, is not easy to dismiss. Unique to this program is a practical and realistic look at the progression of trouble that is experienced by the offender, from one false belief to the next. Call Number: Vid 94, 94.1.

Health Awareness and HIV Risk Reduction Program for Inmates at Correctional Institutions
Health Services Office, Department of Corrections
2 Martin Luther King, Jr., Drive S.E., Room 952
East Floyd Tower
Atlanta, GA 30334
(404) 656–6400 attn.: Joe Geoffrey
The curriculum represents a cooperative effort between the Georgia Department of Corrections and the Georgia Department of Human Resources to provide a risk-reduction educational program for inmates at correctional institutions. All incoming inmates to the state penal system are tested for the HIV antibody and receive basic HIV/AIDS education and ongoing counseling from correctional counselors and medical staff. The curriculum is designed to supplement those efforts.

HIV Resource Library
225 Broadway, 23rd Floor
New York, NY 10007
(212) 693–0995 attn.: Rosa Benedicto
This library has several videos targeted toward prison populations. Individuals must go to the facility to complete their own research. It is not available by phone, fax, or mail.

It's Like This
The HIV Center
722 West 188th St.
New York, NY 10032
(212) 740–0047 attn.: Kenia Fernandez
Video focusing on the impact of HIV on women and their families.

The Meeting
The HIV Center
722 West 188th St.
New York, NY 10032
(212) 740–0047 attn.: Kenia Fernandez
Video of three women and their attitudes toward their own risk for
HIV.

Price of Freedom Is Living Free (Relapse, Recidivism, and Recovery)
Office of Substance Abuse Programs
524 I St.
Sacramento, CA 95814
(916) 327–3707 attn.: Rita A. Norman
Thirty minutes. A practical guide to avoiding relapse and recidivism. This program is an excellent tool to prepare client/inmate
groups for re-introduction into the community. It teaches techniques such as how to practice the H.A.L.T. maneuver (Am I Hun-
gry, Angry, Lonely, or Tired), and how to identify the warning signs
of the relapse process while developing a relapse prevention plan.
Call Number: Vid 59.

*Protecting Yourself from AIDS and Other Infectious Diseases, Instructor's
Guide*
State of New York Department of Health, AIDS Institute
1215 Western Ave., Suite 306
Albany, NY 12203
(518) 431–1218 attn.: Tracy McCumber
A step-by-step lesson plan for conducting in-service training or a
continuing education program on infectious diseases.

Recovery Is an Inside Job
National Council of La Raza: La Raza AIDS Center (NCLR)
Union Station Plaza
810 First St., NE, Suite 300
Washington, D.C. 20002
Frank Beadle, project director

Soap Scenes
722 West 188th St.
New York, NY 10032
(212) 740-0047

Starting Over: Three Ex-Offenders Talk About Living with HIV
State of New York Department of Health, AIDS Institute
1215 Western Ave., Suite 306
Albany, NY 12203
(518) 431–1218 attn.: Tracy McCumber
Target audience is prisoners, parolees, and persons with criminal records.

List of HIV/AIDS Curricula

AIDS, Can I Get It?
Substance Abuse Library Listings
Office of Substance Abuse Program
524 I St.
Sacramento, CA 34283–0001
(916) 327–3707 attn.: Rita Norman
This video provides a better understanding of AIDS risk reduction: the facts about AIDS, how it is transmitted, and how to reduce the risk of becoming infected.

AIDS Counseling and Education Program (ACE)
Bedford Hills Correctional Facility
247 Harris Rd.
Bedford Hills, NY 10507
(914) 241–3100 attn.: Liz Mastriani

AIDS Video Project
Juvenile Court Health Services and JWCH Institute
1925 Daly St., 1st Floor
Los Angeles, CA 90038
(213) 962–1600
Joan Melrod, M.P.H., CHES, project coordinator

Be Good to Yourself: A Self-Care Manual for Inmates Living with HIV
AIDS Project Los Angeles
6721 Romaine St.
Los Angeles, CA 90038
(213) 962–1600

Behavioral and Attitudinal Change Model: HIV/STD Harm Reduction for the Incarcerated Population
Scott Cozza, LCSW, ACSW
73 Mission Dr.
Petaluma, CA 94952
(707) 762–1557
Reports facts about prisons and prisoners and steps for HIV prevention and management.

The Empowerment Program: A Curriculum for Health Education Groups for Women at Rikers Island
Hunter College Center on AIDS, Drugs, and Community Health
425 E. 25th St.
New York, NY 10010–2590
(212) 481–1622
B. E. Richie, author
This manual enables women in the Rikers Island detention facilities to take an active part in reducing their risk of HIV infection.

Health Awareness and HIV Risk Reduction Program for Inmates at Correctional Institutes
Georgia Department of Human Resources
Division of Public Health, Epidemiology, and Prevention Branch
2 Peachtree St., 10th Floor, Room 400
Atlanta, GA 30303
(404) 656–6400; fax (404) 651–6414 attn.: Joe Geoffrey, M.S.W.
This curriculum represents an attempt to provide a risk-reduction education program for inmates at correctional institutions.

HIV/AIDS and Reproductive Health: A Peer Trainer's Guide
Women's Project
2224 Main St.
Little Rock, AR 72206
(501) 372–5113

HIV/AIDS Education and Prevention in Correctional Facilities
Multicultural AIDS Coalition
801B Tremont St.
Boston, MA 02118
(617) 442–1622
Douglass Park, author
This is an outline for a proposed course for incarcerated persons.
The course examines the interrelationships among substance use
and abuse, sexual behavior, and HIV infection.

HIV/AIDS Peer Education Program
Louisiana State Penitentiary at Angola
Box 15258
New Orleans, LA 70175–5258
(504) 899–0619
Shannon E. Hager, R.N., M.P.H., nurse consultant

Just Say Know to AIDS: Safer Sex
Substance Abuse Library Listings
Office of Substance Abuse Program
524 I St.
Sacramento, CA 34283–0001
(916) 327–3707 attn.: Rita Norman
The program includes a series of compelling interviews with HIV-
positive and AIDS patients, who share what it is really like living
with the dying from AIDS.

Lo Que Hizo Ramon [What Ramon Did]
Substance Abuse Library Listings
Office of Substance Abuse Program
524 I St.
Sacramento, CA 34283–0001
(916) 327–3707 attn.: Rita Norman
Created by Hispanics for Hispanics to describe everyone's respon-
sibility to control the spread of AIDS.

Marin AIDS Project
San Quentin State Prison
Center of AIDS Prevention Studies, University of California, San Francisco
1660 Second St., San Rafael, CA 94901
(415) 457–2487 attn.: Barry Zack
Collaborative programs in HIV prevention. Programs include comprehensive peer education: HIV education of new inmates by HIV-positive peer inmate educators and support for newly diagnosed HIV-positive inmates by HIV-positive peer counselors.

Massachusetts Department of Youth Services
Wormwood St., Suite 400
Boston, MA 02210
(617) 727–7575 attn.: Gary Shostak

Oregon AIDS Support Inmate Services (O.A.S.I.S.)
2605 State St.
Salem, OR 97310–0505
(503) 371–6483

The Plan
Substance Abuse Library Listings
Office of Substance Abuse Program
524 I St.
Sacramento, CA 34283–0001
(916) 327–3707 attn.: Rita Norman
This video looks at two individuals who carry the double burden of being HIV infected and addicted.

Power Moves: A Situational Approach to HIV Prevention for High Risk Youth
Rocky Mountain Center for Health Promotion and Education
7525 West 10th Ave.
Lakewood, CA 80215–5141
(303) 239–6494; fax (303) 239–8428

Roger's Story
Substance Abuse Library Listings
Office of Substance Abuse Program
524 I St.
Sacramento, CA 34283–0001
(916) 327–3707 attn.: Rita Norman
Forty-four-year-old Roger shares the harrowing experience of his twenty-year struggle with addiction, his attempts to go straight, and his subsequent diagnosis with AIDS.

So Sad, So Sorry, So What
Substance Abuse Library Listings
Office of Substance Abuse Program
524 I St.
Sacramento, CA 34283–0001
(916) 327–3707 attn.: Rita Norman
A portrait of a single mother, prison inmate, and recovering addict who now has AIDS.

STDs and HIV/AIDS Peer Educators Training Manual: A Complete Guide for Trainers of Peer Educators in the Prevention of STDs Including HIV/AIDS
U.S. Border Health Association
Training and Technical Assistance Project
6060 N. Mesa, Suite 600
El Paso, TX 79912
(915) 581–6645 attn.: Rosa Benedicto
This manual has been designed for use by trainers of peer educators dedicated to STDs and HIV/AIDS prevention. It can be used by trainers from many organizations, including departments of health, government agencies, private volunteer organizations, and nongovernmental and community-based organizations that provide training for outreach workers.

Training and Technical Assistance Project (TTAP) Border AIDS Partnership (BAP)
U.S. Mexico Border Health Association (USMBHA)
6006 N. Mesa, Suite 600
El Paso, Texas 79912
(915) 581–6645; fax (915) 584–8701

Women and AIDS, the Greatest Gamble
Substance Abuse Library Listings
Office of Substance Abuse Program
524 I St.
Sacramento, CA 34283–0001
(916) 327–3707 attn.: Rita Norman
A series of women are interviewed about how they got AIDS.

List of HIV/AIDS Publications

Being Alive
3626 Sunset Blvd.
Los Angeles, CA 90026
(213) 667–3262

Criminalization of the AIDS Epidemic
National Lawyers Guild AIDS Network
55A Capp St.
San Francisco, CA 94110
(415) 285–5066
Article that talks about mandatory testing and AIDS. $2.25.

Critical Path AIDS Project
2062 Lombard St.
Philadelphia, PA 19146
(215) 735–2762

Inmate to Inmate
Gilbert Sarrano
c/o PWA Coalition Newsline
31 W. 26th St., Room 125
New York, NY 10010
(212) 532–0290 or (212) 532–0568
Brochure developed by prisoner addressing AIDS and HIV issues.

National Institute of Justice (NIJ)
National Criminal Justice Reference Service
P. O. Box 6000
Rockville, MD 20849
(800) 851-3420
NIJ publishes reports: *AIDS in Correctional Facilities, AIDS in Proba-tion and Parole Services,* and *HIV/AIDS and STDs in Juvenile Facilities.*

Ryan's Vision
Suite 6-F277 Prospect Ave.
Hackensack, NJ 07601

References

Abt Associates. (1995). Unpublished data.

AIDS Commission. (1991). Prison opportunity is wasted. *Alcoholism and Drug Abuse Week, 3,* 5.

AIDS in Prison Project. (1994). *National policy agenda covering prisoners and former prisoners living with AIDS/HIV in the U.S.* Manuscript submitted for publication.

Airhihenbuwa, C. O. (1989). Perspectives on AIDS in Africa: Strategies for prevention and control. *AIDS Education and Prevention, 1*(1), 57–69.

Airhihenbuwa, C. O., DiClemente, R. J., Wingood, G. M., & Lowe, A. (1992). HIV/AIDS education and prevention among African-Americans: A focus on culture. *AIDS Education and Prevention, 4*(3), 267–276.

Albov, A. P., & Issaev, D. D. (1994). Homosexual contacts among male prison inmates in Russia [Abstract No. 490D]. *International Conference on AIDS, 10*(2), 53.

Allard, F., April, N., Martin, C., Brisson, C., Bergeron, G., Gingras, S., & Paradis, R. (1992). Knowledge and attitudes of correctional facilities staff towards HIV and HBV infections. [Abstract No. PuD 9003]. *International Conference on AIDS, 8*(3), 199.

Altice, F. L. (1994, June). *Discharge planning and continuity of love for HIV infected female inmates.* Paper presented at the Health Resources and Services Administration Conference on Specific Programs of National Significance, Washington, DC.

Anderson v. Murdaugh, No. 1:92–2694–17BD, U.S. District Court of South Carolina (October 25, 1993).

Andrus, J. K., Fleming, D. W., Knox, C., McAlister, R. O., Skeels, M. R., Conrad, R. E., Horan, J. M., & Foster, L. R. (1989). HIV testing in prisoners: Is mandatory testing mandatory? *American Journal of Public Health, 79*(7), 840–842.

Anno, B. J. (1991). *Prison health care: Guidelines for the management of an adequate delivery system.* Washington, DC: National Institute of Corrections.

Applewhite v. *United States,* 614 A.2d 888 (D.C. Cir. 1992).

Arizona v. *John Wayne Ellevan,* 1 CA-CR 93–0754-PR, Ariz. Ct. App., Div One (1993).

Auerbach, J. D., Wypijewska, C., & Brodie, H. K. (1994). *AIDS and behavior: An integrated approach* (executive summary). Washington, DC: National Academy Press.

Baxter, S. (1991). AIDS education in the jail setting. *Crime and Delinquency, 37*(1), 48–63.

Bedford Hills Correctional Facility. (1995). [Brochure]. ACE Office.

Behrendt, C. Kendig, N., Dambita, C., Horman, J., Lawlor, J., & Vlahov, D. (1994). Voluntary testing for human immunodeficiency virus (HIV) in a prison population with a high prevalence of HIV. *American Journal of Epidemiology, 139*(9), 918–926.

Belbot, B. A., & del Carmen, R. (1991). AIDS in prison: Legal issues. *Crime and Delinquency, 37,* 135–153.

Belgrave, F. Z., Randolph, S. M., Carter, C., Braithwaite, N. (1993). The impact of knowledge, norms, and self-efficacy on intentions to engage in AIDS-preventive behaviors among young incarcerated African American males. *Journal of Black Psychology, 19*(2), 155–168.

Berkman, A. (1995). Prison health: The breaking point. *American Journal of Public Health, 85*(12), 1616–1618.

Bernasconi, S., Buechi, M., & Stutz, S. T. (1994). AIDS prevention in a Swiss prison: A pilot project including the distribution of sterile injection equipment [Abstract No. PD0523]. *International Conference on AIDS, 10*(2), 336.

Boudin, K., & Clark, J. (1990). Community of women organize themselves to cope with the AIDS crisis. A case study from Bedford Hills correctional facilities. *Social Justice, 17,* 90–107.

Bowser, B. P. (1986). Community and economic context of black families: A critical review of the literature 1909–1985. *The American Journal of Social Psychiatry, 6*(17), 1–26.

Boyle, B. A., & Kummer, L. H. (1994, June). *Medical case management for correctional systems: The Maryland model for inmates with HIV infection.* Paper prepared for Health Resources and Services Administration Conference on Specific Programs of National Significance, Washington, DC.

Braithwaite, R., & Mayberry, R. (1996). Formative evaluation of HIV/AIDS risk reduction programs in prison settings: Final report (Cooperative Agreement No. SO75-13/14). Washington, DC: Association of Schools of Public Health and Centers for Disease Control and Prevention.

Brewer, T. F., & Derrickson, J. (1992). AIDS in prison: A review of epidemiology and preventive policy. *AIDS, 6*(7), 623–628.

Brewer, T. F., Vlahov, D., Taylor, E., Hall, D., Munoz, A., & Polk, B. F. (1988). Transmission of HIV-1 within a statewide prison system. *AIDS, 2*(5), 363–367.

Brien, P. M., & Harlow, C. W. (1995). *AIDS in the prison, 1993*. Washington, DC: U.S. Department of Justice (NCJ-152765).

Bureau of Justice Statistics. (1993). *Jail inmates 1992*. Washington, DC: U.S. Department of Justice, Author.

Burris, S. (1992, November). Prisons, law, and public health: The case for a coordinated response to epidemic disease behind bars. *University of Miami Law Review, 47*, 291–335.

Bustos, P., Arredondo, A., & Child, R. (1993). HIV/AIDS in prisons—Chile [Abstract No. W5-D11–4]. *International Conference on AIDS, 9*(1), 114.

Calzavara, L. M., Major, C., Myers, T., Schlossberg, J., Millson, M., Wallace, E., Rankin, J. & Fearon, M. (1995). Reducing volunteer bias: Using left-over specimens to estimate rates of HIV infection among inmates in Ontario Canada. *AIDS 9*, 631–637.

Capaldini v. Sheriff of San Francisco County, Cal. App. Ct. 1st Dist., No. A052533 (1991).

Carrell, A.L.M., & Hart, G. J. (1990). Risk behaviors for HIV infection among drug users in prison. *British Medical Journal, 300*, 1383–1384.

Casey v. Lewis, 773 F. Supp. 1365 (D. Ariz. 1991).

Casey v. Lewis, 4 F.3d 1516 (9th Cir. 1993).

Castro, K. G., Conley, L. J., Shansky, R., Scardino, V., Green, T., Narkunas, J., Coe, J., Horsburgh, L. R., & Hammett, T. (1994). *Report of a study of HIV infection in selected Illinois correctional facilities*. Unpublished manuscript.

Celentano, D. D., Brewer, T. F., Sonnega, J., & Vlahov, D. (1990). Maryland inmates' knowledge of HIV-1 transmission and prevention: A comparison with the U.S. general population. *Journal of Prison and Jail Health, 9*, 45–54.

Centers for Disease Control. (1988a). Guidelines for effective school health education to prevent the spread of AIDS. *Morbidity and Mortality Weekly Report, 37*(S-2), 1–14.

Centers for Disease Control (1988b, June). Update: Universal precautions for prevention of transmission of HIV, hepatitis B virus, and other blood-borne pathogens in health care settings. *Morbidity and Mortality Weekly Report, 37*, 377–382.

Centers for Disease Control. (1989, June). Guidelines for prevention of transmission of HIV and hepatitis B virus to health-care and public-safety workers. *Morbidity and Mortality Weekly Report, 38*(25), 446.

Centers for Disease Control (1990). *HIV/AIDS: U.S. AIDS cases reported through July 1990*. Atlanta: Author.

Centers for Disease Control. (1991a). HIV prevention in the U.S. correctional system. *Morbidity and Mortality Report, 41,* 389–397.

Centers for Disease Control. (1991b, June). *HIV/AIDS surveillance report.* Atlanta: Centers for Disease Control, Center for Infectious Diseases, 1–18.

Centers for Disease Control. (1992a). HIV prevention in the U.S. correctional system, 1991. *Morbidity and Mortality Weekly Report, 41*(22), 379–397.

Centers for Disease Control. (1992b). Selected behaviors that increase risk for HIV infection, other sexually transmitted diseases, unintended pregnancy among high school students—United States, 1991. *Morbidity and Mortality Weekly, 41*(50), 945–950.

Centers for Disease Control. (1992c). Unpublished data.

Centers for Disease Control and Prevention. (1993, April 19). *HIV/AIDS Prevention Bulletin.*

Centers for Disease Control and Prevention. (1994a). Health risk behaviors among adolescents who do and do not attend school—United States, 1992. *Morbidity and Mortality Weekly, 43*(8), 129–132.

Centers for Disease Control and Prevention. (1994b, September). HIV/AIDS surveillance report. *Morbidity and Mortality Weekly Report, 9*(9), 1–5.

Centers for Disease Control and Prevention. (1995). Trends in sexual risk behavior among high school students—United States, 1990, 1991, and 1993. *Morbidity and Mortality Weekly Report, 44*(7), 124–132.

Chalk v. U.S. District Court Central District of California, 840 F.2d 701 (9th Cir. 1988).

Chesney, M. A., & Folkman, S. (1994). Psychological impact of HIV disease and implications for intervention. *Psychiatric Clinics of North America, 17*(1), 163–182.

Cohen, D., Scribner, R., Clark J., & Cory D. (1992, April). The potential role of custody facilities in controlling sexually transmitted diseases. *American Journal of Public Health, 82*(4), 552–556.

Confidentiality said breached by serving food on paper plates. (1990, December 12). *AIDS Policy and Law,* p. 3.

Connor v. Foster, 833 F. Supp. 727 (N.D. Ill. 1993).

Correctional Association of New York AIDS in Prison Project (1994). *Draft for a national policy agenda concerning prisoners and former prisoners living with AIDS/HIV in the United States.* Unpublished manuscript.

Cozza, S. (1994). *Behavioral and attitudinal change model: HIV/STD harm reduction for the incarcerated population* [Curriculum]. HIV/AIDS Peer Education Program, State Medical Facility for Prisoners. P.O. Box 2000, Vacaville, CA 95695–2000.

de Jongh-Wieth, F. E., & Schepp-Beelen, J. C. (1994). Promoting safe behavior in prison: A program directed at detainees and prison staff [Abstract No. PC0345]. *International Conference on AIDS, 10*(2), 246.

De Wit, J. (1994). AIDS in prison in Belgium. In P. A. Thomas & M. Moerings (Eds.), *AIDS in prison* (pp. 74–83). Brookfield, VT: Dartmouth Publishing.

Derby v. *Allison,* Civil No. 4–93-CV-10160 (S.D. Iowa 1993/1996).

Des Jarlais, D. C., Padian, N. S., & Winkelstein, W., Jr. (1994). Targeted HIV-prevention programs. *New England Journal of Medicine, 331*(21), 1451–1453.

Diamond, J. (1994). HIV testing in prison: What's the controversy? (letter). *Lancet, 344*(8938), 1605–1651.

DiClemente, R. J., Lanier, M. M., Horan, P. F., & Lodico, M. (1991). Comparison of AIDS knowledge, attitudes, and behaviors among incarcerated adolescents and a public school sample in San Francisco. *American Journal of Public Health, 81*(5), 628–630.

District of Columbia. (1992, June 12). Inmate lacks standing to request HIV-based segregation. *AIDS Litigation Reporter,* p. 8244.

Dixon, P. S., Flanigan, T. P., DeBuono, B. A., Laurie, J. J., De Ciantis, M. L., Hoy, J., Stein, M., Scott, H. D., & Carpenter, C.C.J. (1993). Infection with the human immunodeficiency virus in prisoners: Meeting the health care challenge (Review). *American Journal of Medicine, 95*(6), 629–635.

Doe v. *City of New York,* 15 F.3d 264 (2d Cir. 1994).

Doe v. *Meachum,* 126 F.D.R. 444 (D. Conn. 1989).

Doe v. *State of New York,* 558 N.Y.S.2d 698 (1992).

Doe v. *Wigginton,* 21 F.3d 733 (6th Cir. 1994).

Dogwood Center. (1995). *Health emergency: The spread of drug-related AIDS among African Americans and Latinos.* Princeton, NJ: Dawn Day.

Dolan, K., Hall, W., Wodak, A., & Gaughwin, M. (1994). Evidence of HIV transmission in an Australian prison. *Medical Journal of Australia, 160*(11), 734.

Dolan, K., Kaplan, E., Wodak, A., Hall, W., & Gaughwin, M. (1994, August). *Modeling HIV transmission in the New South Wales prisons, Australia.* Poster abstract PD0524 presented at the International Conference on AIDS, Yokohama.

Doll, D. C. (1988, January). Tattooing in prison and HIV infection. *Lancet, 1*(8575–6), 66–67.

Dolley, M. (1995). Denmark opinion is divided. *British Medical Journal, 310,* 280.

Donaldson, S. (1994). *Rape of incarcerated males in the USA: A preliminary statistical look* (5th ed.). Unpublished manuscript.

Dorozynski, A. (1995). France: One in five prisoners rejects voluntary HIV test. *British Medical Journal, 310,* 281.

Dubler, N. N., & Sidel, V. W. (1989). On research on HIV infection and AIDS in correctional institutions. *Milbank Quarterly, 67*(2), 171–207.

Dumond, R. W. (1992). The sexual assault of male inmates in incarcerated settings. *International Journal of the Sociology of Law, 20,* 135–157.

Dunn v. *White,* 880 F.2d 1188 (10th Cir., 1989), *cert. denied* 110 S. Ct. 871 (1990).

Emslie, J., Taylor, A., Goldberg, D., Wrench, J., & Gruer, L. (1994). HIV outbreak in a Scottish prison: Intervention [Abstract No. PD0526]. *International Conference on AIDS, 10*(2), 337.

Estelle v. *Gamble,* 429 U.S. 97; 97 S.Ct. 285 (1976).

Expert Committee on AIDS and Prisons. (1994, February). *HIV/AIDS in prisons: Final report of the expert committee on AIDS and prisons.* Montreal: McGill Centre for Ethics, Medicine, and Law.

Farmer v. *Brennan,* 114 S.Ct. 1970 (1994).

Farmer v. *Moritsugu,* 742 F.Supp 525 (W.D. Wisc. 1990).

Feest, J. & Stover, H. (1994). AIDS in prisons in Germany. In P. A. Thomas & M. Moerings (Eds.), *AIDS in prison* (pp. 20–29). Brookfield, VT: Dartmouth Publishing.

Flanigan, T., Bury-Maynard, D., Vigilante, K., Burzynsky, J., Bubly, G., Kim, J., Rich, J., Zierler, S., DeCiantis, M., Normandy, L., Snead, M., De Groot, A., Loberti, P., DeBuono. B. (1995). *The Rhode Island prison release program: Progress and challenges in linking incarcerated individuals with HIV/AIDS to community services.* Washington, DC: U.S. Department of Health and Human Services, Health Resources Services Administration.

Flanigan, T., Kim, J., Zierler, S., Rich, J., Vigilante, K., Bury-Maynard, D. (1996, June). A prison release program for HIV-positive women linking them to health services and community follow-up (letter). *American Journal of Public Health, 86*(6), 886–887.

Florida Department of Corrections. (1993, February 23). Taking the mystery out of HIV prevention, testing, and treatment. (Video teleconference).

Florio, S., Bellini, E., Safyer, S., Fletcher, D. (1992). *HIV infection in New York City jails: A voluntary program.* Poster abstract POC 4318 presented at the VIII International Conference on AIDS, Amsterdam.

Friedman, S., Quimby, E., Sufian, M., Abdul-Quader, A., & Des Jarlais, D. C. (1988, Winter/Summer). Racial aspects of the AIDS epidemic. *California Sociologist,* pp. 55–68.

Gates v. *Deukmejian,* CIVSW 87–1636 (E.D. California 1990), settlement approved March 8, 1990.

Gates v. *Rowland,* No. 93–15363, 93–16136, D.C. No. CV-87–01636-LKK (9th Cir. 1994), opinion dated November 4, 1994.

Gaughwin, M. D., Douglas, R. M., Davies, L., Mylvaganam A., Liew, C., & Ali R. (1990). Preventing human immunodeficiency virus (HIV) infection among prisoners: Prisoners' and prison officers' knowledge of HIV and their attitudes to options for prevention. *Community Health Studies, 14*(1), 61–64.

Gellert, G. A., Maxwell, R. M., Higgins, K. V., Pendergast, T., & Wilker, N. (1993). HIV infection in the women's jail, Orange County, California, 1985 through 1991. *American Journal of Public Health, 83*(10), 1454–1456.

Gerlel, Z., Szlavik, J., Banhegyi, D., & Miskovits, E. (1994). Knowledge and attitude to HIV/AIDS in Hungarian garrisons and prisons [Abstract No. PC0346]. *International Conference on AIDS, 10*(2), 246.

Gillies, P., & Carballo, M. (1990). Adult perception of risk, risk behaviour, and HIV/AIDS: A focus for intervention and research. *AIDS, 4,* 943–951.

Givens, T. (1994, October). *Leaving the penitentiary with HIV infection.* Paper presented at HIV/AIDS Prevention Conference, Louisiana State Penitentiary, Angola, LA.

Glaser, J. B., & Greifinger, R. B. (1993). Correctional health care: A public health opportunity (Review). *Annals of Internal Medicine, 118*(2), 139–145.

Glick v. *Henderson,* 855 F.2d 536 (8th Cir. 1988).

Gostin, L. O. (1992, Fall). The Americans with disabilities act and the U.S. health care system. *Health Affairs, 11*(3), 248–257.

Greenberg, R., & Halperin, S. (1994, November). *Early intervention services for HIV infected inmates.* Paper presentation at 122nd annual meeting and exhibition of the American Public Health Association, Washington, DC.

Greenspan, J. (1994). Struggle for compassion: The fight for quality care to women with AIDS at central California's women's facility. *Yale Journal of Law and Feminism, 6,* 383–395.

Hammett, T. M. (1994, May 23). *Rape and HIV/AIDS in prisons: District problems requiring different policy responses.* Testimony before the joint committee on public safety, general court of Massachusetts.

Hammett, T. M., Harrold, L., Gross, M., & Epstein, J. (1994). *1992 update: HIV/AIDS in correctional facilities: Issues and options.* U.S. Department of Justice, Washington, D.C.

Hammett, T. M., & Widom, R. (1996). HIV/AIDS education and prevention programs for adults in prisons and jails and juveniles in confinement facilities—United States, 1994. *Morbidity and Mortality Weekly Report, 45*(13), 268–271.

Hammett, T. M., Widom, R., Epstein, J., Gross, M., Sifre, S., & Enos, T. (1995). *1994 Update: HIV/AIDS and STDs in correctional facilities.* Washington, DC: U.S. Department of Justice, National Institute of Justice, and U.S. Department of Health and Human Services, Centers for Disease Control and Prevention.

Harding, T. W. (1987, November). AIDS in prison. *Lancet, 2*(8570), 1260–1263.

Harding, T. (1995). HIV infection in prisons: What about the WHO guidelines? *British Medical Journal, 310*(6989), 1265.

Harlow, C. W. (1993). *HIV in U.S. prisons and jails.* Annapolis Junction, MD: Bureau of Justice Statistics Clearinghouse.

Harm Reduction Coalition. (1995). *Working together towards individual and community health* [Brochure]. Alan Lithographer, Inc.

Harris v. Thigpen, 727 F.Supp. 1564 (M.D. Alabama 1990).

Harris v. Thigpen, 941 F.2d 1495 (11th Cir. 1991).

HIV Peer Education Program. (1993). Together we can make a difference. [Brochure, author S. Cozza]. Vacaville, CA: Vacaville Medical Facility,

Horsburgh, C. R., Jarvis, J. Q., McArther, T., Ignacio, T., Stock, P. (1990). Seroconversion to HIV in prison inmates. *American Journal of Public Health, 80*(2), 209–210.

Howleit, T., & Stauffer, K. (1994, June). *Progress and challenges in linking incarcerated individuals with HIV/AIDS to community services.* Paper presented at the Health Resources and Services Administration Special Programs of National Significance Conference, Washington, DC.

Hu, D. J., Keller, R., & Fleming, D. (1989). Communicating AIDS information to Hispanics: The importance of language and media preference. *American Journal of Preventive Medicine, 5*(4), 196–200.

Hutchinson, J. (1992). AIDS and racism in America. *Journal of the National Medical Association, 84*(2), 119–124.

Ibrahim, I. A. (1994). *An assessment of AIDS/HIV knowledge, attitudes, and risk behaviors among parole violators and new commitments to the Virginia Department of Corrections, 1994.* Richmond: Virginia Commonwealth University, Survey Research Laboratory, Center for Public Service.

Illinois appeals court overrules state on testing of prisoner who bit guard. (1994, August 19). *AIDS Policy and Law,* 2–3.

Illinois Compiled Statutes, 410, 305/7(c) (1992).

Inmates of New York with Human Immunodeficiency Virus v. Cuomo, No. 90-CV-252 (N.D. N.Y. 1990).

Jaccard, J., Turrisi, R., & Wan, C. K. (1990). Implications of behavioral decision theory and social marketing for designing social action programs. In J. Edwards, R. S. Tindale, L. Heath, & E. J. Posavac (Eds.),

Social influence processes and prevention (pp. 103–142). New York: Plenum Press.

Jimenez, R. (1987, November). Educating minorities about AIDS: Challenges and strategies. *Family and Community Health, 10*(3), 70–73.

Johnetta v. *Municipal Court,* 218 Cal. App. 3d 1255 (1990).

Johnson v. *United States,* 816 F.Supp 1519 (N.D. Ala. 1993).

Joseph, A. (1994, October). *The impact of life sentences on HIV/AIDS in prison.* Paper presented at the meeting of the HIV/AIDS Prevention Conference, Louisiana State Penitentiary, Angola, LA.

Jurgens, R. (1994a). AIDS in prisons in Canada. In P. A. Thomas & M. Moerings (Eds.), *AIDS in Prison* (p. 134). Aldershot, UK: Dartmouth Press.

Jurgens, R. (1994b). HIV prevention taken seriously: Provision of free syringes in a Swiss prison. *Canadian HIV/AIDS Policy and Law Newsletter, 1*(1), 1–3.

Jurgens, R., Gilmore, N., & Richard, C. (1993). HIV/AIDS and prisons: Making necessary changes possible [Abstract No. PO-D12–3691]. *International Conference on AIDS, 9*(2), 833.

Kamerman, J. (1991). Corrections officers and acquired immune deficiency syndrome: Balancing professional distance and personal involvement. *Death Studies, 15*(4), 375–384.

Karches, H. L. (1995). Germany: Approach varies widely between states. *British Medical Journal, 310,* 282.

Kendig, N., Stough, T., Austin, P., Kummer, L., Swetz A., & Vlahov, D. (1994). Profile of HIV seropositive inmates diagnosed in Maryland's state correctional system. *Public Health Reports, 109*(6), 756–760.

Knight-Ridder, H. M. (1994, July 29). Sentencing differences for crack, powder cocaine affect African Americans. *Boston Globe,* p. 0792.

Konner, M. (1993). *Medicine at the crossroads.* New York: Pantheon.

LaChance-McCullough, M. L., Tesoriero, J. M., Sorin, M. D., & Lee, C. (1993). Correlates of HIV seroprevalence among male New York state prison inmates: Results from the New York state AIDS institute criminal justice initiative. *Journal of Prison and Jail Health, 12,* 103–134.

LaChance-McCullough, M. L., Tesoriero, J. M., Sorin, M. D., & Stern, A. (1994). HIV infection among New York state female inmates: Preliminary results of a voluntary counseling and testing program. *The Prison Journal, 73*(2), 198–215.

Lanier, M. M., DiClemente, R. J., & Horan, P. F. (1991). HIV knowledge and behaviors of incarcerated youth: A comparison of high and low risk locales. *Journal of Criminal Justice, 19,* 257–262.

Lanier, M. M., & McCarthy, B. R. (1989). AIDS awareness and the impact of AIDS education in juvenile corrections. *Criminal Justice Behavior,* *16,* 395–411.

Lile v. *Tippecanoe County Jail,* 844 F.Supp. 1301 (N.D. Ind. 1992).

Lurigio, A. J., Petraitis, J., & Johnson B. R. (1991, January). HIV education for probation officers: An implementation and evaluation program. *Crime and Delinquency, 37,* 125–134.

Lurigio, A. J., Petraitis, J., & Johnson, B. R. (1992). Joining the front line against HIV: An education program for adult probationers. *AIDS Education and Prevention, 4,* 205–218.

Macher, A. (1994, June). *Access to continuity of care for inmates with HIV disease: The federal initiative.* Paper prepared for Health Resources and Services Administration Conference on Specific Programs of National Significance, Washington, DC.

Machon, S., Lopez, S., & Meletiche, S. (1994). What to do leaving prison if you are HIV. *PWA Support* [newsletter of Prisoners Legal Services of New York], *6,* 1–3.

Magis, C., Del Rio, A., Gonzalez, G., Garcia, M. L., Valdespino, J. L., & Sepulveda, J. (1994). HIV infection in prison in Mexico. *International Conference on AIDS, 10*(2), 44.

Magura, S., Kang, S.-Y., & Shapiro, J. L. (1994). Outcomes of intensive AIDS education for male adolescent drug users in jail. *Journal of Adolescent Health, 15*(6), 457–463.

Magura, S., Kang, S.-Y., Shapiro, J., & O'Day, J. (1993). HIV risk among women injecting drug users who are in jail. *Addiction, 88*(10), 1351–1360.

Mahaffey, K. J., & Marcus, D. K. (1995). Correctional officers' attitudes toward AIDS. *Criminal Justice and Behavior, 22*(2), 91–105.

Mahon, N. (1994a, August). *Let's talk about sex and drugs: HIV transmission and prevention behind bars.* Abstract PD0521 presented at the 10th International Conference on AIDS, Yokohama.

Mahon, N. (1994b, November). *Peer education and counseling in New York city and state correctional facilities.* Paper presented at the American Public Health Association Annual Meeting, Washington.

Mays, V. M., & Cochran, S. D. (1988). Issues in the perception of AIDS risk and risk reduction activities by black and Hispanic/Latina women. *American Psychologist, 43*(11), 949–956.

McDonald, D. C. (1994, September). *Managing prison health care and costs.* Manuscript submitted for publication.

McKee, K. J., Markova, I., & Power, K. G. (1995). Concern, perceived risk and attitudes towards HIV/AIDS in Scottish prisons. *AIDS Care, 7*(2), 159–170.

McKee, K. J., & Power, K. G. (1992). HIV/AIDS in prisons. *Scottish Medical Journal, 37*(5), 132–137.

Miller, H., Turner, C., & Moses, L. (1990). *AIDS: The second decade.* Washington, DC: National Academy Press.

Miller, J. G. (1995, August 10). Comment. *The New York Times* (on-line).

Moerings, M. (1994). AIDS in prisons in the Netherlands. In P. A. Thomas & M. Moerings (Eds.), *AIDS in prison* (pp. 56–73). Brookfield, VT: Dartmouth Publishing.

Moody v. *Daggett,* 429 U.S. 78 (1976).

Moritsugu, K. (1993, March). *Communicable disease crisis: Corrections and the community.* Presentation conducted at meeting sponsored by American Correctional Health Services Association and the Centers for Disease Control and Prevention, Atlanta.

Morris, R. E., Baker, C. J., & Huscroft, S. (1992). Incarcerated youth at risk for HIV infection. In R. J. DiClemente (Ed.), *Adolescents and AIDS: A generation in jeopardy* (pp. 52–69). Thousand Oaks, CA: Sage Publications.

Morse, D. L., Truman, B. I., Hanrahan, J. P., Mikl, J., Broaddus, R. K., Maguire, B. H., Grabau, J. C., Kain-Hyde, S., Han, Y., & Lawrence, C. E. (1990, March). AIDS behind bars: Epidemiology of New York state prison inmate cases, 1980–1988. *New York State Journal of Medicine, 90*(3), 133–138.

Mudur, M. (1995). India: Campaigners urge check on spread of HIV. *British Medical Journal, 310,* 280.

Muhammad v. *Federal Bureau of Prisons,* D. DC No. 91–3244 [CRR]. (1991, opinion dated April 1992).

Mutter, R. C., Grimes, R. M., & Labarthe, D. (1994). Evidence of intraprison spread of HIV infection. *Archives of Internal Medicine, 154*(7), 793–795.

Myers v. *Maryland Division of Correction,* 782 F.Supp. 1095 (D. Md. 1992).

Nader, P. R., Wexler, D. B., Patterson, T. L., McKusick L., & Coates, T. (1989). Comparison of beliefs about AIDS among urban, suburban, incarcerated, and gay adolescents. *Journal of Adolescent Health Care, 10,* 413–418.

National Commission on AIDS. (1991, March). *Report: HIV disease in correctional facilities.* Washington, DC: U.S. Government Printing Office.

Nelles, J., & Harding, T. (1995). Preventing HIV transmission in prison: A tale of medical disobedience and Swiss pragmatism. *Lancet, 346*(8989), 1507–1508.

New hope for medical parole. (1994, Summer/Fall). *PWA Support* [newsletter of Prisoners Legal Services of New York], *6,* pp. 7, 10.

New Jersey v. *Smith,* N.J. Super. Ct., App. Div., No. A-636389-T4 (1993).

New York v. *Larson,* N.Y. App. Div, 1st Dept. (1993).

New York v. *Rios,* N.Y. Sup. Ct., Kings Co., No. SCI5626/92 (January 19, 1993).

Nolley v. *County of Erie,* 776 F.Supp. 715 (W.D. N.Y. 1991).

Normand, J., Vlahov, D, & Moses, L. E. (Eds.). (1995). *Preventing HIV transmission: The role of sterile needles and bleach.* Washington, DC: National Academy Press.

Nyamathi, A. & Shin, D. M. (1990). Designing a culturally sensitive AIDS educational program for black and Hispanic women of childbearing age. *NAACOGS Clinical Issues in Perinatal and Women's Health Nursing, 1*(1), 86–98.

Occupational Safety and Health Administration (OSHA). (1994). Occupational exposure to bloodborne pathogens. 29 *Code of Federal Regulations* 1910.1030, December 6, 1991.

Oliveira, S., & Longo, P. (1993). Projeto tereza: New strategies for HIV/AIDS prevention among prisoners [Abstract No. PO-D12–3696]. *International Conference on AIDS, 9*(2), 834.

Olivero, J. M. (1990). The treatment of AIDS behind the walls of correctional facilities. *Social Justice, 17*(1), 113–125.

Oregon AIDS Support (Inmate) Services. (1994, September). *Annual Report.* Available from O.A.S.I.S., 2605 State Street, Salem OR 97310–0505.

Ormond v. *Mississippi,* Miss. Sup. Ct. No. 89-KA-0221 (1989).

Pagliaro, L. A., & Pagliaro, A. M. (1992, April). Sentenced to death? HIV infection and AIDS in prisons—current and future concerns. *Canadian Journal of Criminology, 34*(2), 201–214.

Peterson, J. L., & Marin, G. (1988). Issues in the prevention of AIDS among black and Hispanic men. *American Psychologist, 43*(11), 871–877.

Platek, M. (1994). AIDS in prison in Poland. In P. A. Thomas & M. Moerings (Eds.), *AIDS in prison* (pp. 30–38). Brookfield, VT: Dartmouth Publishing.

Polonsky, S., Kerr, S., Harris, B., Gaiter, J., Fichtner, R. R., & Kennedy, M. G. (1994). HIV prevention in prisons and jails: Obstacles and opportunities. *Public Health Reports, 109*(5), 615–625.

Pont, J., Strutz, H., Kahl, W., & Salzner, G. (1994). HIV epidemiology and risk behavior promoting HIV transmission in Austrian prisons. *European Journal of Epidemiology, 10*(3), 285–289.

Power, K. G., Markov, I., Rowlands, A., McKee, K. J., & Kilfelder, C. (1991a). Inmates' self-perceived risk of HIV infection inside and outside Scottish prisons. *Health Education Research, 9*(1), 47–55.

Power, K. G., Markov, I., Rowlands, A., McKee, K. J., Anslow, P. J., & Kilfelder, C. (1991b). Sexual behaviors in Scottish prisons. *British Medical Journal, 302,* 1507–1508.

Prisons' care systems swamped by AIDS epidemic, panel told. (1990, December 12). *AIDS Policy and Law,* p. 3.

Rickman, R. L., Lodico, M., DiClemente, R. J., Morris, R., Baker, C., & Huscroft, S. (1994). Sexual communication is associated with condom use by sexually active incarcerated adolescents. *Journal of Adolescent Health, 15,* 383–388.

Rogers, D. E., & Osborn, J. E. (1993). AIDS policy: Two divisive issues. *Journal of the American Medical Association, 270*(4), 494–495.

Rogers, M. F., & Williams, W. W. (1987, Spring). AIDS in blacks and Hispanics: Implications for prevention. *Issues in Science and Technology,* pp. 89–94.

Rolf, J., Nanda, J., Baldwin, J., & [Author needed]. (1991). Substance misuse and HIV/AIDS risks among delinquents: A prevention challenge. *International Journal of Addictions, 25,* 533–559.

Room, R. (1974, Fall). Minimizing alcohol problems. *Alcohol, Health and Research World,* 12–17.

Rotily, M., Galinier-Pujol, A., Obadia, Y., Moatti, J. P., Toubiana, P., Vernay-Vaisse, & Gastaut, J. A. (1994). HIV testing, HIV infection, and associated risk factors among inmates in south-eastern French prisons. *AIDS, 8*(9), 1341–1344.

Schaller, G. (1993). WHO guidelines on HIV/AIDS in prisons: A comparison between the 1987 and 1992 versions [Abstract No. WS-D11–6]. *International Conference on AIDS, 9*(1), 114.

Scherdin, L. (1994). AIDS in prisons in Norway. In P. A. Thomas & M. Moerings (Eds.), *AIDS in prison* (pp. 7–19). Brookfield, VT: Dartmouth Publishing.

Schilling, R., el-Bassel, N., Ivanoff, A., Gilbert, L., Su, K. H., & Safyer, S. M. (1994). Sexual risk behavior of incarcerated, drug-using women, 1992. *Public Health Reports, 109*(4), 539–547.

Schlichtman, B. S. (1994, October 9). Peer plan curbs AIDS at Angola. *Baton Rouge Sunday Advocate.*

School Board of Nassau County v. *Arline,* 480 U.S. 272 (1987).

Selwyn, P. (1987). Issues for drug treatment and public health. *Advances in Alcohol and Substance Abuse, 7*(2), 99–105.

Sennott, C. M. (1994a, May 1–3). Rape behind bars. *Boston Globe,* pp. 1, 18, 19 (May 1); pp. 1, 6 (May 2); pp. 1, 6 (May 3).

Sennott, C. M. (1994b, Nov. 9). Prison system enacts reforms to stop inmate rape. *Boston Globe,* pp. 37–43.

Sheldon, T. (1995). Netherlands: Potential HIV epidemic feared in jails. *British Medical Journal, 310,* 281.

Siegal, D. M. (1992). Rape in prison and AIDS: A challenge for the eighth amendment framework of *Wilson* v. *Seiter. Stanford Law Review, 44,* 1541, 1551–1552.

Siegel-Itzkovich, J. (1995). Israel: All prisoners have voluntary HIV test. *British Medical Journal, 310,* 283.

Singer, M. (1991). Confronting the AIDS epidemic among IV drug users: Does ethnic culture matter? *AIDS Education and Prevention, 3*(3), 258–283.

Smith, P. F., Mikl, J., Truman, B. I., Lessner, L., Lehman, J. S., Stevens, R. W., Lord, E. A., Broaddus, R. K., & Morse, D. L. (1991). HIV infection among women entering the New York state correctional system. *American Journal of Public Health, 81,* 35–40.

Snider, D. E., Thorburn, R. C., Warren, R. C., & Dowdle, W. R. (1993). *Correctional health care: A neglected public health opportunity.* Manuscript submitted for publication.

State v. *Farmer,* 805 P.2d 200 (Washington, 1991).

Stevens, J., Zierler, S., Cram, V., Dean, D., Mayer, K. H., & De Groot, A. S. (in press). Risks for HIV infection in incarcerated women. *Journal of Women's Health.*

Sudman, S., & Bradburn, N. M. (1974). *Response effects in surveys: A review and synthesis.* Chicago: Aldine.

Sullivan, L. W. (1989). Shattuck lecture—the health care priorities of the Bush administration. *New England Journal of Medicine, 321*(2), 125–128.

Taylor, A., Goldberg, D., Emslie, J., Wrench, J., Gruer, L., Cameron, S., Black, J., Davis, B., McGregor, J., Follett, E., Harvey, J., Basson, J., & McGavigan, J. (1995). Outbreak of HIV infection in a Scottish prison. *British Medical Journal, 310*(6975), 289–292.

Thomas, P. A. (1994). AIDS in prisons in England and Wales. In P. A. Thomas & M. Moerings (Eds.), *AIDS in prison* (pp. 39–55). Brookfield, VT: Dartmouth Publishing.

Thomas, P. A., & Moerings, M. (Eds.). (1994). *AIDS in prison* (Introduction). Aldershot, UK: Dartmouth Press.

Thomas, S., & Quinn, S. (1991). The Tuskegee syphilis study 1932–1972: Implications for HIV education and AIDS risk reduction programs in the black community. *American Journal of Public Health, 81*(11), 1498–1505.

Townsey, R. D. (1981). The incarceration of black men. In L. E. Gary (Ed.), *Black men* (pp. 229–256). Thousand Oaks, CA: Sage Publications.

Turnbull, P. J., & Dolan, K. A. (1992). *Prison decreases the prevalence of behaviors but increases the risk.* Poster abstract POC4321 presented at the VIII International Conference on AIDS, Amsterdam.

Turnbull, P. J., Dolan, K. A., & Stimson, G. V. (1993). HIV testing and the care and treatment of HIV-positive people in English prisons. *AIDS Care, 5*(2), 199–206.

Turnbull, P. J., Stimson, G. V., & Stilwell, G. (1994). *Drug use in prisons.* Horsham, West Sussex, UK: AIDS Education and Research Trust.

Turner v. *Safley,* 482 U.S. 78, 107 S.Ct. 2254 (1987).

U.S. General Accounting Office (1991). *Drug treatment: State prisons face challenges in providing services.* (AGAD/HRD-91–128). Report to the Committee on Government Operations.

Valdiserri, E. V., Hartl, A. J., & Chambliss, C. A. (1988). Practices reported by incarcerated drug abusers to reduce risk of AIDS. *Hospital and Community Psychiatry, 39*(9), 966–972.

Vaz, R. G., Gloyd, S., Folgosa, E., & Kreiss, J. (1995). Syphilis and HIV infection among prisoners in Maputo, Mozambique. *International Journal of STD and AIDS, 6*(1), 42–46.

Virginia v. *Webb,* No. F-796–93, Petersburg (Va.) Cir. Ct. (1994).

Vlahov, D., Brewer, F., Munoz, A., Hall, D., Taylor, E., & Polk, B. F. (1989). Temporal trends of human immunodeficiency virus type 1 (HIV-1) infection among inmates entering a statewide prison system, 1985–1987. *Journal of Acquired Immune Deficiency Syndromes, 2*(3), 283–290.

Vlahov, D., Brewer, T. F., Castro, K. G., Narkunas, J. P, Salive, M. E., Ullrich, J., & Muñoz, A. (1991). Prevalence of antibody to HIV-1 among entrants to U.S. correctional facilities. *Journal of the American Medical Association, 265*(9), 1129–1132.

Vumbaca, G. (1994). Effective HIV/AIDS policies and programs for the prison system [Abstract No. 488D]. *International Conference on AIDS, 10*(2), 53.

Walker, J. (1992). AIDS update. *The National Prison Project Journal, 7*(4), 26.

Walker v. *Sumner,* 917 F.2d 382 (9th Cir. 1990).

Weaver v. *Reagan,* 8th Cir., No. 88–2560, Slip opinion (September 25, 1989); *affirming,* W.D. Mo., No. 87–4314-CV-C-5 (September 29, 1988).

Weeks v. *Collins,* D.C. S. Tex., S. Div. No. 93–3708 (October 11, 1994).

Weeks v. *Morales,* D.C. S. Tex., S. Div. No. H-93–3708 (1993).

Weeks v. *Scott,* 55 F.2d 1059 (5th Cir. 1995).

Weeks v. *State of Texas,* 834 S.W.2d 559 (1992).

Weisbuch, J. B. (1991). The new responsibility for prison health: Working with the public health community. *Journal of Prison and Jail Health, 10*(1), 3–18.

Weisfuse, I. B., Greenberg, B. L., Back, S. D., Makki, H. A., Thomas, P., Rooney, W. C., & Rautenberg, E. L. (1991). HIV-1 infection among New York City inmates. *AIDS, 5*(91), 1133–1138.

Wexler, H. K., Magura, S., Beardsley, M. M., & Josepher, H. (1994). ARRIVE: An AIDS education/relapse prevention model for high-risk parolees. *International Journal of Addiction, 29*(3), 361–386.

Widom, R., & Hammett, T. M. (1996). *Research in brief: HIV/AIDS and STDs in juvenile facilities.* Washington, DC: National Institute of Justice.

Wilson v. Seiter, 501 U.S. 294, 111 S.Ct. 2321 (1991).

Witherspoon, G. A. (1994, October). *HIV/AIDS double impact—workable solution.* Paper presented at HIV/AIDS Prevention Conference, Louisiana State Penitentiary, Angola, LA.

World Health Organization. (1993, March). *WHO guidelines on HIV infection and AIDS in prison.* Geneva, Swit.: Global Programme on AIDS.

Zimmerman, S. E., Martin, R., & Vlahov, D. (1991). AIDS knowledge and risk perceptions among Pennsylvania prisoners. *Journal of Criminal Justice, 19,* 239–256.

Index